Bernard Neugeboren, PhD

Environmental Practice in the Human Services: Integration of Micro and Macro Roles, Skills, and Contexts

Pre-publication
REVIEWS,
COMMENTARIES,
EVALUATIONS . . .

" **I**n this pathbreaking book that identifies practice skills that can be used in direct-service, community, and policy settings, Neugeboren challenges social work faculty to move beyond people changing to environmental practice."

Bruce S. Jansson, PhD
Professor,
School of Social Work,
University of Southern California

More pre-publication
REVIEWS, COMMENTARIES, EVALUATIONS . . .

"**T**his is a well-organized text, written by a well-organized, experienced, knowledgeable teacher well-versed in the subject matter. Each chapter begins with a table of contents, a case history that is woven into the text, a summary, and a study-discussion guide. It is practical and readable, usable by students in social work, community psychology, rehabilitation, and public health. An obvious labor of love, it evidences many years of experience, concern, thought, and teaching. The student will find concrete help.

The book focuses on the person and environment in a unique, revelatory way better than any other comparable text known to this reviewer. It moves seamlessly from micro to macro and back. It has revolutionary potential. It overflows with thoughtful, provocative analyses and suggestions. The literature review is superb.

It aims to redirect much of the intervention effort from the individual psychosocial to the social ecological, informing the reader how and why. It focuses on system, not individual modifications. It targets the two intervention systems as potentially cooperative, not necessar-

ily conflicting. Neugeboren focuses on the superordinate goal of serving the consumer/client."

Harold W. Demone, Jr., PhD
Professor II Emeritus and Former Dean,
School of Social Work,
Rutgers University;
Visiting Lecturer in Health Policy
and Management,
Harvard School of Public Health

"**P**rofessor Neugeboren's latest book, *Environmental Practice in the Human Services*, is an authoritative discussion of what is needed for social workers to engage in truly generic practice. Professor Neugeboren offers a much-needed corrective to the current emphasis of professional social workers on providing clinical services with little or no regard to the organizational and environmental impact on their clients' situations. Since the days of the settlement houses in the late nineteenth century, there has always been a dimension of social work practice that stresses environmental influences over individual factors as critical to understanding the causes of social problems. Neugeboren's text is clearly part of that historical tradition, as well as being responsive to the current movement in social work education to integrate the various types of social work practice (i.e., casework, community work, administration) into a generalist practice model.

Environmental Practice in the Human Services is a comprehensive, well-documented, and highly readable text. The author presents a model of environmental practice followed by an extensive and detailed discussion of the kinds of micro and macro practice skills that are needed to implement this model. The author then shows how environmental practice works in a number of areas, with special emphasis on its role in providing services to individuals with chronic problems. This book will serve as a valuable text in courses on micro/macro social work practice, and other approaches to generalist practice."

Burton Gummer, PhD
Professor, School of Social Welfare,
Nelson A. Rockefeller College
of Public Affairs and Policy,
University at Albany

"**N**eugeboren presents a powerful old/new proposal for social environmental practice, by bringing together an enormous body of social work literature, from the early days of the profession, to the most recent studies by Jack Rothman, David Mechanic, Harry Specht, and others. He seeks to facilitate change in individuals' problematic situations as well as changes in policies related to social problems through modification of the social contexts, rather than personal changes, as is currently so popular in our psychiatrically and medically oriented society. This is especially clear in the case of extremely vulnerable people (such as the severely disabled) for whom 'cure' is not possible, whereas environmental support and stimulation may enhance quality of life.

However, the importance of the book emerges when social environmental practices are viewed as relevant to and within ordinary micro and macro social contexts. Here, Neugeboren's fundamental premise emerges: Social environmental practices involve a wide array of activities that enable people's 'natural capacity to adapt given a benevolent environment.' The book consists of a systematic presentation of methods and approaches to create and to coordinate such benevolent environments at the organizational, community, and societal levels.

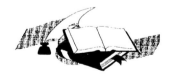

Through case illustrations and citations, Neugenboren demonstrates these to be social work's historic mission—and its future."

Martin Bloom, PhD
Professor,
School of Social Work,
University of Connecticut

"**T**his book may be the most ambitious attempt yet to conceptualize an environmental praxis for social work. For much of this century, the profession has struggled with incorporating environmental interventions into its core technology. Notwithstanding the general acceptance of the person-environment paradigm, relatively little progress has been made in operationalizing the skills and knowledge social workers in direct practice would need to change the environmental circumstances of consumers. Drawing on macro theory and practice research in social work and related fields, e.g., community psychology, Neugeboren does a commendable job of organizing and synthesizing what is known about intervening in agency, community, and policy environments to modify noxious environmental forces and increase access to resources. Perhaps more important, he has provided specific guidelines and case examples that give concrete dimension to this technology. Armed with these specific skills, direct-service practitioners will be better able to work with the severely disabled and frail populations that increasingly comprise agency caseloads.

While developing the technology of environmental intervention is a first step to practice applications, it will not be sufficient unless agency policies and incentive structures are modified to support this kind of practice. Neugeboren is alert to the essential interdependence of technology and organizational context and provides important insights into how the latter must be changed to enable the former.

Overall this is a much-needed book that arrives at a time when social work is trying to find a fit between its historic mission, fashioned in the early twentieth century, and current realities. At least one answer seems to lie in finding a way to link the micro and macro practice perspectives. Neugeboren has made an important contribution to forging this link."

Rino Patti, DSW
Professor and Dean,
School of Social Work,
University of Southern California

Environmental Practice in the Human Services

Integration of Micro and Macro Roles, Skills, and Contexts

HAWORTH Social Work Practice
Carlton E. Munson, DSW, Senior Editor

New, Recent, and Forthcoming Titles:

Environmental Practice in the Human Services

Integration of
Micro and Macro Roles,
Skills, and Contexts

Bernard Neugeboren, PhD

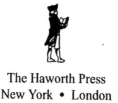

The Haworth Press
New York • London

© 1996 by The Haworth Press, Inc. All rights reserved. No part of this work may be reproduced or utilized in any form or by any means, electronic or mechanical, including photocopying, microfilm and recording, or by any information storage and retrieval system, without permission in writing from the publisher. Printed in the United States of America.

The Haworth Press, Inc., 10 Alice Street, Binghamton, NY 13904-1580

Library of Congress Cataloging-in-Publication Data

Neugeboren, Bernard.
    Environmental practice in the human services : integration of micro and macro roles, skills, and contexts / Bernard Neugeboren.
        p.   cm.
    Includes bibliographical references and index.
    ISBN 0-7890-6025-6 (alk. paper).
    1. Human services. 2. Social service. 3. Social ecology. I. Title.
HV31.N47 1995
361–dc20   95-25071
                                                                              CIP

This book is dedicated to Ramona and Anna and to all others who have the strength of character and moral commitment to assume personal responsibility for caring for those who are vulnerable.

ABOUT THE AUTHOR

Bernard Neugeboren, PhD, is Professor at the Rutgers University School of Social Work where he initiated and developed a masters program in social work administration and has taught since 1967. A specialist in social work administration, mental health, and organizational theory, Professor Neugeboren has done research on organizational behavior and field education in social work administration. His articles have appeared in *Administration in Social Work, Journal of Sociology and Social Welfare, Social Work, Journal of Aging Social Policy, Psychosocial Rehabilitation Journal,* and *Journal of Education for Social Work.* He is author of the books *Psychiatric Clinics: A Typology of Service Patterns* and *Organization, Policy and Practice in the Human Services* and is currently working on his fourth book, *Community-Based Generalist Practice.*

CONTENTS

PART II. ENVIRONMENTAL PRACTICE IN ACTION

Acknowledgments

I am indebted to my wife, Ramona Neugeboren, who developed and implemented an environmentally oriented community-based model for public child welfare services in New Jersey that is the source of the administrative content in macro community resource coordination (Chapter 5). This environmentally oriented service-delivery model is discussed in "Psychological Work To Social Work" (Neugeboren 1991:305-313). Witnessing my wife's effort to improve the welfare of severely disabled children and adults and the mentally ill has reenforced my belief in the efficacy of environmental practice in the human services.

I also wish to thank Robert Morris, former professor at the Florence Heller Graduate School of Social Welfare, for the influence he had on my interest in environmental practice, in part through his seminal article on social care (Morris 1977). Harold Demone and Uri Aviram provided constructive criticism that helped stimulate my conceptualization of environmental practice. Charles Garvin was the most helpful with editorial assistance. Also appreciated is the secretarial support provided by Betty McCoy, Gloria Johnson, and Suzanne Orsogna, as well as the technical computer assistance I received from the staff at the Rutgers Computer Center. The educational leave provided by Rutgers University through Dean Mary Davidson was instrumental in allowing time to complete this book. Finally, I would like to acknowledge staff members of The Haworth Press: William Palmer, Managing Editor; Susan Trzeciak, Production Editor; Dawn Krisko, Production Editor; Peg Marr, Senior Production Editor; Marylouise Doyle, Cover Design Director; and Lillian Rodberg, the indexer. They were most helpful in efficiently expediting the publication of this book.

Foreword

The concept of a social work practice that concentrates on environmental matters, as defined in this new text, is a promising and valuable step in the evolution of the still-novice profession of social work that has been evolving and changing over the past 90 years. The significance of this volume is that it may open the way to recapturing the conceptual breadth that characterized, more latently than explicitly, the first 40 years of social work as a professional as well as occupational entity. This recapturing will involve substantial shifts in thinking about what constitutes the self-proclaimed profession and what kind of education foundation it will require.

Social work education, and practices, have long wrestled with the issue of nature versus nurture. It chose for its core concept the intersection of person and society—the problems of individuals as they mature and cope with living within a widening circle of influences, from the relationships within a family, to the neighborhood, to the local institutions of community and society. These provide the psychological as well as the social environments (care, values, affection, conflict, socialization, income, shelter, informal learning, education for skills, occupation, and acceptance or rejection) that give individuals the capacities to cope with life's adult realities. Some understanding of each and all is necessary for a profession that deals with disfunctional individuals and groups. Such an ambitious task has proven difficult to realize.

In the early years, the field developed two main institutional tracks to cover the spectrum—the family casework agency concerned with individuals, families, and children, and the settlement house (later the group work and/or community organization agency) concerned with the economic/social environment and how individuals working in groups can modify that environment. There were specialized professional social worker associations and courses of study either in comprehensive schools or in specialized ones which chose one or the other focus. Examples include Smith College with its early behavioral concentration; Simmons College for medical; and the YMCA/YWCA schools or Universities of Pittsburgh and Western Reserve University, known for community organization or group work.

By the 1990s the situation was quite different. The field had flourished in the growth years of 1940 to 1975; university-based graduate and undergraduate education proliferated. The specialty associations were replaced by a unified professional association that slowly developed a standard formula for membership. The career and job market began to split into two areas in the 1930s: the mass public income programs with large resources and staffs requiring administration and organization skills, and the private family or child care agencies and mental health agencies that emphasized skills in psychological and individual or family interrelationships. The educational system was oriented to the latter. In the 1920s it adopted the Flexner model of medical education. This model required a university base for basic scientific study plus a university link to practice agencies (such as hospitals) for learning and for experimentation, and was influenced by traditional academic disciplines.

The accrediting agency for schools of social work, trying to adapt the medical model to the special concerns of social work, ended up adopting a uniform prototype curriculum for all social work training. That prototype in time concentrated heavily on learning borrowed and adapted from psychiatry, psychology, and sociology theories. The career opportunities and jobs in mental health and counselling, and financing for graduate study (via National Institute of Mental Health grants and stipends), all provided the incentives for that concentration. The mass public income agencies accepted the credentialling of the profession for promotion to many public positions but the numbers of openings appealing to social workers was insufficient to alter the character of the training.

In fairness, the profession tried valiantly to accommodate to other than behavioral careers. However, there were constraining factors. First, schools were straightjacketed by a maximum of two years for study at the MSW level with part of that time usually devoted to apprentice or internship placements in service agencies. Here teaching and supervisory staffs were—with a few exceptions—only tenuously identified with the university academic environment. The continuum from baccalaureate study was most loose. The demand for more and more interpersonal competence by employing agencies plus the preference of students for counselling careers combined to pre-empt most of the available teaching time. The counter pressure to introduce more and more information about a variety of social and economic problems consumed most of the remaining curricular space. Little time was left to teach or learn intensively about other methods for social workers to deal with the social environment—once known as community planning or organization. Second, in an expanding era, there was insufficient interest among advocates to train social workers for such functions, especially when the nation had sufficient organizational specialists recognized for competence in organization, administration, and planning, albeit in fields other than social work—public administration, public health, urban planning, economics, etc.

One of the minor factors that may have hampered social worker attempts to secure support was the predisposition to advocate for more basic changes in society than were acceptable to the larger public, such as proposals for income redistribution that involved major changes in the economic structure, and the addition of representatives of workers, the poor, and political liberals to central decision making in agency boards.

The social work solution was to adopt a mandatory generic education base to fit within its resource limits; however, the generic was heavily weighted by psychological thinking, scanting other approaches. Until recently it was unable to break out of these constraints.

The political and economic environment of the 1990s, and for the decade ahead, is in the midst of major change in the structure of social welfare. In such an era the appearance of this volume is timely. Painful and difficult changes lie ahead if the promise of this text is to be realized. The author has identified well many of the social issues that social workers confront. To treat them effectively will also require development of methods suitable for the magnitude of the tasks. It will necessitate the evolution of methods comparable to those experienced by the schools in the past 40 years as they built the dominating position of interpersonal theory and methods into the curricular space with minor space for elaboration of social environmental or social organizational skills. With hope we can anticipate a gradual alteration in the allocation of that curricular space, either in all schools, or more likely in a few pioneering schools which can secure accreditation waivers. Such a trend may allow time for some social workers to acquire new skills to expand the qualified teaching pool. (The Brandeis experiments begun in 1959 were such an effort to move some attention from casework to policy and planning.) Alternatively the field may replicate what the interpersonal and counselling elements of the field did: borrow physicians, psychiatrists, and psychologists in the 1930s and 1940s who were not social workers but who were willing to transfer some of their skills to social workers who then adapted them for social work.

The main theses of this text are well-suited for adoption in existing schools of social work. If the larger, longer-term prospect is to be realized–to restore parity between social/economic environmental and the interpersonal psychological careers which social work concepts once embraced–the basic teaching text needs to be followed by efforts to overcome accumulated obstacles. The next step may be to see if, and how, scattered interests in such an evolution among professionals in the field can be consolidated.

Robert Morris
Professor Emeritus
Brandeis University

Preface

Public concern for the physical environment, stimulated in the 1960s by the popular book *Greening of America* (Reich 1970), led to the enactment of the National Environmental Policy Act of 1969 and the subsequent creation of the federal department of the Environmental Protection Agency. Activists promoted "Earth days" to publicize the need to preserve our natural environment, and the federal government responded with legislation ensuring clean air and water, as well as pesticide, waste, and noise control.

New developments in the social and behavior sciences reflect these concerns with the physical environment. Architects and city planners focus on the organization of urban centers and new towns. Human ecologists and geographers analyze ways that communities adapt and grow. Psychologists and sociologists design environments to maximize individual functioning and competence. Psychiatrists and social workers identify ways that social environments facilitate the handling of life crises (Moos 1976). Thus, the social movement to protect the physical environment stimulated renewed emphasis within the human services on the importance of enhancing *social environments*. In their early history, the helping professions put much emphasis on "environmental manipulation" as a basic mission. Social reform efforts of such pioneers as Dorothea Dix and Jane Addams drew attention to the negative impact of dysfunctional environments such as slum housing, sweatshop work conditions, or dehumanizing mental institutions. Although state licensing has given renewed impetus and legitimation to private psychotherapeutic practice (40 percent of social work professionals are in private practice serving the middle-class), there is also increasing interest in viewing the "person in the environment" (Specht and Courtney 1994:4). The "ecological" perspective in social work emphasizes the impact of social environment on service consumers (Germain and Gitterman 1980). Pressure to give more attention to environmental interventions increases as society recognizes that there are substantial numbers of people with severe disabilities who cannot be cured but who can benefit from more benevolent environments. There is realization that approaches developed for acute, short-term problems may not be appropriate for the needs of highly vulnerable populations (Rothman 1994). This book on environmental practice is to rectify in a small way the historical imbalance in the human services toward an emphasis on people-changing methods, giving secondary emphasis to environmental change. It moves beyond the more general conceptual emphasis in the current literature on person-in-environment toward the development of an environmental practice technology based on an intervention model which prescribes specific micro and macro roles and functions.

THEMES OF THE BOOK

There are four major themes encompassed in this book: (1) the need to return human services to the historic mission of environmental change; (2) the influence of organizational contexts on practice; (3) the similarities, differences, and interdependencies between micro and macro practice; and (4) the appropriateness of environmental practice for highly vulnerable populations.

Historic Mission of Environmental Change

The overall goal of this book is to point to the need for the human services to return to their historic mission of environmental change (Specht and Courtney 1994). Environmental change is operationalized on the micro level as changing situations for individual service consumers and on the macro level as modification of program policies and structures. Environmental practice seeks to remedy the overemphasis in the human services on changing the attitudes and behaviors of service users through clinical intervention. It attends to the environmental component of the person/environment relationship assuming that situational change in itself can be sufficient for accomplishment of service consumer benefit. Although environmental change can be beneficial to all service users, it is an especially appropriate intervention for highly vulnerable populations.

Organizational Contexts of Practice

A second theme of this book is that organizational contexts affect the opportunities and constraints of professional interventions. These emanate from the goals and structures of the agencies where practice occurs. The conceptual framework developed here for environmental practice (see Chapter 2) acknowledges that interventions will vary depending on whether they occur in one of three practice arenas: organizational, community, or societal. The organizational arena includes direct service agencies; the community arena consists of social advocacy and social planning organizations; and the societal arena is comprised of policy formulating agencies (e.g., legislature). The differences in goals and structures of these sponsoring organizations affect the intervention roles that can be assumed in each of these different practice settings. For example, there are greater constrains on performing social advocacy in direct service agencies than in agencies that have this function as their primary goal (e.g., citizen committees on children, mentally ill, etc.).

The impact of organizational context depends on whether practice occurs on the micro or macro level, as well as on the specific role the practitioners perform. Roles establish boundaries for professional behavior, prescribing opportunities and limits on action. The objective of *micro* practice is to *change situations* for individuals and groups of service users. Micro practice typically occurs in the roles of direct-service worker and community organizer. The goal of *macro* interventions is to *change policies.* Macro practice distinctively arises in the roles of administrator, social planner, and policy analyst. These organizationally defined roles provide the sanctions and limits for the varying types of environmental practice. For example, direct service people are constrained in their efforts to change agency policies because their role does not provide the sanction (power) and support necessary to engage in this kind of activity. In contrast, the definition of the administrator's role provides the power to change or develop policies.

Organizational context is a basic feature of the conceptual framework used in this book. It is reflected in a two-dimensional model combining practice arenas with micro and macro levels of intervention. The focus is on professional roles that exist in current practice.

Understanding the impact of organizational context is essential for effective practice. Knowing the opportunities and constraints on professional actions arising from different contexts facilitates a more efficient use of resources, since energies can be used to exploit opportunities rather than wasted in attempts to overcome constraints that cannot be modified.

Similarities, Differences, and Interdependencies Between Micro and Macro Practice

Another major theme of this book is the assumption that there are both similarities and differences between micro and macro practice, as well as, interdependencies and linkages between these two intervention levels.

Similarities and Differences Between Micro and Macro Practice

The model of environmental practice used here assumes that micro and macro interventions share a common knowledge base and skills. Common conceptual knowledge is derived from social structural, interorganizational exchange, bureaucratic, and systems theories. Common environmental practice skills include decision making, monitoring, leadership, representing, negotiating, and staffing. Although the technical aspects of these skills are similar, their use will vary depending on whether the practitioner seeks to change service user situations or change policies. Differences occur also because of the variations among arenas of practice (e.g., organizational, community, societal). Different practice contexts require different applications of the skills generic to both levels of practice. As a result, leadership can occur on all levels of the agency. However, different opportunities and constraints are present within the upper and lower organizational levels. Some assume that leadership is possible only at the upper organizational levels. However, the opposite may be the case where executives have less knowledge of the direct-service practice issues than the caseworker who has information derived from contact with service users. This expert power of the caseworker will facilitate his/ her leadership. These environmental practice skills are discussed in Chapter 3.

Interdependencies Between Micro and Macro Practice

Relations between micro and macro practitioners is often laden with tension associated with power, control, and professional autonomy (Neugeboren 1991:136-137). However, this potential for conflict is lessened by the interdependence between these two levels of practice. Micro and macro practice interdependencies arise from shared goals of consumer benefit and the need for communication to obtain information required by both levels of service. Feedback from micro to macro levels is needed by administrators, planners, and policymakers to change ineffective policies. Micro practitioners need information from macro staff about the rationale of policies designed to enhance consumer benefit. Micro staff are also dependent on macro staff for the authority and support required to do their work.

Environmental Practice with Vulnerable Populations

A fourth theme of this book is that environmental interventions are particularly appropriate for highly vulnerable populations, such as the severely mentally and physically ill, the developmentally disabled, and the frail elderly. Although environmental practice can be useful for service consumers with acute problems, it is especially suitable for severely disabled service users who cannot be "cured," but who can benefit from benevolent environments. The chronic nature of the problems suffered by the severely disabled also poses severe demands on the family, necessitating service strategies that provide them with support and assistance.

CONTENTS OF BOOK

Part I: Introduction and Framework for Environmental Practice

Part I introduces environmental practice by discussing the historical antecedents and a conceptual framework for this kind of practice.

Chapter 1 introduces the *need* for environmental practice in conjunction with the *history* of past efforts to develop this emphasis in the human services.

Chapter 2 presents a framework for an environmental practice technology. It is based on practice on the micro and macro levels and in three practice arenas: direct-service agencies, community planning and social advocacy organizations, and social policy formulating agencies.

Part II: Environmental Practice in Action

Part II consists of the application of environmental practice to several areas of human service intervention: community resource coordination; social support; the organizational environment; and practice with highly vulnerable populations. Six practice skills are integrated with these areas.

Chapter 3 indicates how *practice skills* operate in environmental practice. Six practice skills common to micro and macro practice are reviewed. They are decision making, monitoring, leadership, staffing, negotiating, and representing. These skills are discussed in terms of how they occur in the three arenas of practice; the technical aspects of these skills; and situational influences affecting the application of these skills in practice. The interrelationship between these six skills in actual practice is also considered.

Chapters 4 and 5 address community resource coordination on the micro and macro levels. Chapter 4 discusses *community resource coordination on the micro level* as a basic function in service provision for vulnerable populations. The coordination of resources is seen as an essential component of a service-delivery model designed to meet the multiple needs of the severely disabled. This intervention model for community resource coordination includes three stages: (1) selecting the appropriate resource; (2) arranging for the service user's utilization of the resource; and (3) supporting the service consumer's utilization of the resource. This is a service user-driven model, placing much emphasis on consumers' ability to identify their needs and wants.

Chapter 5, discusses *community resource coordination on the macro level,* supplementing the content on micro level coordination in Chapter 4. Emphasis is on the interdependency between micro and macro resource coordination based on the need for macro support to facilitate case coordination and feedback from the micro practitioner on the need for policy change.

Chapters 6 and 7 move into another area of environmental practice particularly relevant for vulnerable populations and their families—social support. Chapter 6 discusses *social support on the micro level*, focusing on its use in serving individual service users. Social support is divided into three areas: mutual aid, self-help, and community support. Four targets of social support— service users, informal caregivers, formal caregivers, and the community at large—are discussed. Social support micro interventions are directed at direct-service agencies, as well as the community organization arena.

Chapter 7 supplements the previous chapter with a presentation of *social support on the macro level*, discussing interventions in direct-service agencies by administrators; in the community arena by social planners; and in the societal arena by policy analysts. The importance of integrating micro and macro social support is also discussed.

Chapter 8 deals with environmental practice in *organizational environments*, and examines how this context influences service effectiveness. An organizational environment model consisting of five areas (physical environment, behavior settings, organizational structure, organizational climate, and organizational culture) is defined and applied to interventions in the organizational, community, and societal arenas of practice.

Chapter 9 discusses environmental practice with *highly vulnerable populations*, focusing on long-term disability as a characteristic of the severely disabled. The trajectory model developed for service to the chronically physically ill is applied to highly vulnerable populations in general and used in environmental interventions in the organizational, community, and societal arenas of practice.

Finally, Chapter 10 discusses some of the implications that environmental practice has for the delivery of human services including the need for specialized education and redistribution of resources in the human-service system.

APPLICATION OF PRINCIPLES OF ENVIRONMENTAL PRACTICE TO CASE SITUATIONS

This book facilitates the application of theories of environmental practice to practice situations by including case material in each chapter. These cases illustrate service problems with the mentally ill, frail elderly, and abused children, depicting environmental interventions on the micro and macro levels in the three arenas of practice. The case material is used to illustrate how the principles, policies, and intervention practices operate in action though application to concrete case situations.

PART I:
INTRODUCTION AND FRAMEWORK
FOR ENVIRONMENTAL PRACTICE

Chapter 1

ENVIRONMENTAL PRACTICE
IN THE HUMAN SERVICES

Environmental Practice
in the Human Services

THE NEED FOR ENVIRONMENTAL PRACTICE

Human-service practitioners, whether they provide direct service to consumers or carry out policy, planning, or administration, are compelled to consider the basic policy question of whether intervention should help individuals to adapt to their situation or whether the problem is embedded in a dysfunctional environment that requires modification. In case practice, assessments are made as to whether the individual's capacities are deficient and need to be enhanced or whether external factors should receive priority. If both factors are operating, which often is the case, time and resource limitations, as well as philosophical orientation, require practitioners to make the difficult decision of whether intervention should focus on the individual or the environment.

Garbarino et al. (1980:9) crystallized the importance of the environmental context in child maltreatment, urging that solutions "must go beyond individualistic therapies and rehabilitation techniques to embrace personal social networks, neighborhoods, and communities." The question for practitioners and policymakers is not simply one of:

> How can we cure the individual pathology of a particular parent? It is also, How can we eradicate the pathology of particular environments? How can we foster environments (or "ecologies") that will relieve the social isolation of families . . . What can our government–local, state and national–do to ensure that people are not isolated from natural networks and that such networks are nurtured rather than undermined by official actions? (9)

Specht and Courtney (1994) also emphasizes the environment in defining the purpose of social work:

> The major function of social work is concerned with helping people perform their normal life tasks by providing information and knowledge, social support, social skills, and social opportunities; it is also concerned with helping people deal with interference and abuse from other individuals and groups,

with physical and mental disabilities, and with overburdening responsibilities for others. (26)

Community planners, policymakers, and administrators of direct-service agencies also need to determine where the primary cause of social problems lie, in the person and/or in the environment. Policy analysts formulating legislative initiatives and guides for direct service programs are required to establish the basis for social policy formulation in terms of programs to change individuals/and or their environments. Community planners who assess community needs and allocate funds to direct-service agencies also need to understand the cause of social problems: is it in the person and/or the situation? Administrators of direct-service agencies, in their tasks of formulating goals, designing structures, and implementing programs, make decisions with the knowledge of the differential cause of service consumers' problems in terms of the individual and/or the environment.

HISTORY OF ENVIRONMENTAL PRACTICE IN THE HUMAN SERVICES

Throughout the history of the human services, varying attention have been given to interventions to change environments. Morris (1986) traces the evolution of "caring for the stranger" from biblical times, noting that American social policy has been somewhat ambivalent about acceptance of communal responsibility for the less fortunate. He observes that in 1980s there was a sharp break with past concern for the disadvantaged.

> Welfare becomes a proxy term for values, a lightning rod for differing views about the obligations we owe each other, the virtues of selfishness, the limits of obligation, and political behaviors, which will either unify or further divide a multiethnic population. (p. 4)

In 1995, with the Republicans gaining control of the Congress, control of welfare policy is shifting from the national to state government through block grants. Whether this will result in decreased public commitment to the needy has yet to be determined. It is our opinion that decentralization of welfare policy to the states may be beneficial in the long run to service consumers since local authorities are compelled to meet unmet social needs because they impact on the quality of life for *all* citizens. This increase of communal responsibility could have implications for a greater emphasis on environmental practice.

The profession of social work has long claimed both expertise as well as societal mandate to achieve "environmental manipulation" for service user benefit. Thus, focus on the environment in social casework practice can be traced back to the very origins of the field (Richmond 1922:99-107). However, the commitment of early casework practice to "external" factors has been questioned (Schriver 1987). Brieland (1990) contrasts the individualistic philosophy (with its "moral means test") of the Charity Organization Society, with which Mary Richmond was identified, with the environmental focus of the settlement house movement represented by Jane Addams. Germain (1994:39-40) cites an incident of Mary Richmond's outraged reaction to Abraham Flexner's address in 1915, "Is Social Work a Profession?", because he stated it was not a profession because it lacked transmissible knowledge and skill of its own, although it did provide a service by connecting people with resources. It is the position of the author that the knowledge and skill required for environmental practice is complex and comparable to that included in other professions.

Although environmental change as a focus for direct practice has received some renewed consideration in recent years (Austin 1986:35-36; Germain and Gitterman 1980; Glasser and Garvin 1977; Grinnell and Kyte 1974; Grinnell 1973; Meyer 1987; Parsons, Hernandez, and Jorgensen 1988), there continues to be primary stress on individual change models in social work practice (Austin and Patti 1984; Grinnell 1973; Meyer 1987:404; Proctor, Voster, and Sirles 1993), as well as in social work education (Ephross and Reisch 1982:280; Gibelman 1983; Schwartz 1977; Lister 1987). The interests of social work students in working with nonchronic middle-class service users is consistent with the emphasis of practice and education (Butler 1990; Rubin and Johnson 1984).

The "medicalization" of the problem of the mentally ill (Aviram 1990:71) and the elderly (Azzarto 1992) is another example of individualizing a social problem, thereby obviating the view that it is affected by structural factors. This disparity between belief and practice relates to the tendency of American social policy to view personal problems as personal failures (Wilensky and Lebeaux 1958). Corrective efforts are therefore directed at individual competence and emotional capacity, even in public welfare programs (Grinnell and Kyte 1975; Teare 1981:100).

One explanation of the lack of development of environmental practice is the failure to appreciate that individual abilities may be less important than situational effects. This is illustrated in research on the factors that predict vocational functioning of the psychiatrically disabled. Anthony and Jansen (1984) found that such individual characteristics as psychiatric symptoms, psychiatric diagnosis, intelligence, and aptitude and personality tests do not predict vocational performance. Also, a patient's functioning in one environment (e.g., community setting) did not predict a person's ability to function in other settings (e.g., work or hospital). In another example, mentally ill persons living in sheltered care were healthier than those living in institutions or in the community (Segal, Vandervort, and Liése 1993). It can be inferred that these different environmental situations were more important than the individual characteristics of the service consumers. Thus, one's situation can be a powerful determinant of social functioning, requiring environmental interventions.

The lack of consistent development of human-service practice focused on changing environments, particularly on the micro level, may also have been due to the lack of a systematic framework for analyzing dysfunctional environments (Austin and Patti 1984:4). In contrast with the more fully developed individual-change models of intervention, frameworks for environmental change have been somewhat general (Brower 1988:411; Garvin and Seabury 1984:4; Harrison 1987:399; Wells and Singer 1985:319), leading to difficulty in operationalizing them in practice. The ecological perspective developed by Germain (1973) provides a broad conceptual framework for environmental practice, but is not in itself a practice model (Germain 1994:41).

Efforts to develop integrated models of practice for changing both the individual and the situation (*person in environment*) may have been unduly influenced by the more highly developed individual-change models (Harrison 1989:73). For example, in the Person-In-Environment (PIE) Scale (Karls and Wandrei 1994), three of the four factors included in the instrument (Factor I–Social Role Problems; Factor II–Environmental Problems; Factor III–Mental Disorders; Factor IV–Physical Disorders) focus on individual dysfunction, while only one factor is concerned with the environment. Generic or integrated models of practice have hindered the field from seeing the differences and inter-relationships between micro and macro practice. The differences between these different intervention levels are evident in actual practice. A theme of this book is to explicate the similarities and differences between micro and macro practice.

The movement in social work education to generalist practice, which is evident in the Council on Social Work Education (CSWE) accrediting standards for bachelor's and master's education (Curriculum Policy Statement 1992), has further impacted on the need for integration of micro and macro practice. A recent proliferation of generalist practice textbooks (Johnson 1995; Kirst-Ashman and Hull 1993; Miley, O'Melia, and DuBois 1995; Tolson, Reid, and Garvin 1994) points to efforts to develop this broader view of practice. However, examination of these texts in terms of the relative amount of content in micro and macro arenas of practice indicates that there is still a primary emphasis on the direct service level of intervention.

Another reason that the theories, tasks, and skills relevant to environmental change have not been applied to the micro level of practice is the lack of transfer of relevant theories and techniques from the macro arena (Abel and Kazmerski 1994:64). The traditional separation between clinical services and the administrative, planning, and social policy areas of education and practice has perpetuated this problem. Macro faculty and practitioners devote their attention primarily to system change efforts because they have not seen the direct practice arena as relevant for their areas of interest and expertise. For example, the exchange theories and techniques applicable to intraorganizational and interorganizational coordination have not been adapted to the micro level linkage of service consumers with resources. System theory on the social environment (Martin and

O'Connor 1989) needs to be operationalized into concrete intervention roles and tasks. The conceptual model of environmental practice used in this book focuses on specific roles and skills.

EFFORTS TO DEVELOP ENVIRONMENTAL PRACTICE

Nevertheless, there were and are efforts to conceptualize and implement micro level environmentally oriented practice. The poverty programs in the 1960s included "environmental therapies" that emphasized "brokerage" and "advocacy" techniques for interventions in community systems on behalf of service users (Gilbert, Miller, and Specht 1980:85-90). Martin Rein (1970) formulated a framework that included radical casework and social policy, which are relevant to micro and macro environmental practice. The model presents a four-cell matrix, with one dimension focus on changing individuals vs. social conditions and a second dimension concentrating on challenging existing standards of behavior. Radical casework is defined as challenging existing behavior standards on an individual level, while radical social policy focuses on changing social conditions. Walz, Willenberg, and DeMoll (1974) proposed that knowledge of environmental design could provide a new dimension to enhance social work services to service consumers.

An example of environmental practice in a poverty program was the Community Progress Inc., which emphasized "opening opportunities" for the poor in three community systems of housing, employment, and education (living, learning, and working environments) (Neugeboren 1970b). Emphasis on "opportunity structures" was derived from sociological deviance theory (Cloward 1959), which led to social service offices in public housing developments, employment training centers, and community schools to ensure that the lower-income groups would have access to social opportunities to facilitate upward social mobility. Intervention into living and work environments is also evident in the Family Support Act of 1988 (Family Support Act 1988), which provides for support services to welfare service users in public housing and employment training.

In the 1980s, there is evidence of increasing attention to environmental practice. For example, in two 1985 issues of *Social Work* there were eight articles dealing with this arena, including social support and self help. Neugeboren (1991:268-286) identified 11 areas of environmental practice, including: social ecology; social provision; resource systems; community support systems; least restrictive environment; normalization; habilitation; open opportunity structures; people processing; discharge planning; and case management. Specht (1985) advocated greater emphasis on techniques for influencing the situation in direct interventions with attention to structural factors. Austin (1986:35) suggests that transferring the macro practice skills to the domain of micro practice "could enhance the abilities of clinicians to engage in environmental interventions." Kruzick and Friesen (1984) specify the community and organizational aspects of serving the severely mentally ill in the community. Berger and Nash (1984) identify macro practice skills in the delivery of hospital social services.

Interest in environmental interventions is linked with social work practice in occupational settings (Balgopal 1989). Industrial organizations have discovered that they can impact positively on the health of their employees by restructuring the work environment (Blair et al. 1986). Live for Life, a program developed in Johnson & Johnson (Wilbur 1983), found that by promoting such programs as fitness, weight control, nutrition, stress management, smoking cessation, and other health promotion efforts, their costs for health insurance were lowered (Bly, Jones, and Richardon 1986).

An experiment on weight reduction from the Live for Life program illustrates the impact of restructuring work environment. Three groups of employees were involved in the experiment: a group that participated in the weight reduction program; a similar group that did not participate but worked in the same building where the weight reduction program took place; and a third equivalent group that also did not participate in the special program but worked in another building. It was found that the group participating in the program lost the most weight; the group that worked in the same building also lost weight; and the third group that worked in another building was unaffected. The explanation for the second group losing weight was the effect that the work environment had on attitudes toward the importance of weight control (e.g., the presence of scales throughout the building).

Although there have been continuing efforts to conceptualize and operationalize social work interventions in the environmental arena, full advantage has not been taken of the knowledge available in allied social science fields of environmental and community psychology. It is believed that the operationalizing of environmental concepts for purposes of empirical study done in these fields holds much promise for formulating environmental strategies and techniques (Walz, Willenberg, and DeMoll 1974:45). This chapter reviews some of this knowledge, with subsequent chapters specifying in depth various areas of environmental practice.

A case situation is first presented to illustrate the concepts discussed. Several environmental practice issues are presented along with a conceptual framework for this type of practice. This framework is subsequently applied to the various environmental practice areas discussed in later chapters. The model includes micro and macro practice levels, as well as three practice arenas: organizational, community, and societal. The various roles and functions performed in these arenas are elaborated. The integration of micro and macro practice is also discussed. Six environmental practice skills will then be defined and further elaborated on in Chapter 3. The chapter concludes with study questions posing practice problems on the micro and macro levels.

CASE: CHILD ABUSE

The Agency

The State Child Protection Agency provides protective services for children to prevent child abuse and support enhancement of family life. The families served are from low-income and minority groups. The agency provides such services as supervision of children in their own homes, day care, homemakers, residential and foster home placement, transportation, and linkage to other community programs such as housing, health, and mental health services.

The Family

The Smith family was referred to the agency by the public school because of suspicion that Mary Jane, age 8, was being physically abused. Mary Jane displayed behaviorial difficulties at school and was not able to keep up with her work. The teacher, Ms. Jones, considered Mary Jane to be "slow," even though testing indicated that she had average intelligence. Mary Jane was placed in a special class for slow learners.

The Smith family consists of the mother, age 35, and four children: a son, age 14; Mary Jane; and two other daughters, ages 4 and 2. The mother's boyfriend, Mr. Henry, lives with the family and is the father of the two younger daughters. Mrs. Smith was deserted by her husband shortly after the birth of Mary Jane. Mr. Smith, who is also the father of the boy, provides sporadic financial support for his two children. Mr. Henry also gives some economic support for the family, but it is limited since he earns minimum wage as a kitchen worker in a restaurant. Although the maternal grandmother lives nearby, her contacts are limited because of conflict with Mr. Henry.

Evaluation of the family situation revealed that the mother was overwhelmed by a multitude of problems. This included lack of adequate income, a crowded living situation, and chronic health problems of family members that went untreated. Mrs. Smith suffered from diabetes and the 14-year-old son was addicted to crack.

Practice in Direct-Service

Investigation by the agency worker confirmed that Mary Jane was being physically abused by the mother's boyfriend. He resented Mary Jane, feeling that she was arrogant and would not respond to his discipline because he was not her father.

The worker, who had an MSW in casework, developed a plan to reduce the abuse of Mary Jane by engaging the mother, the boyfriend, and Mary Jane in individual counseling, with a focus on the problems in the relationship between Mary Jane and Mr. Henry. The worker believed that the abuse problem could be dealt with by intensive counseling over a relatively short time period that would result in prevention of abuse in the future. This would also help Mrs. Smith to develop the ability to remedy her situation including finding better housing and dealing with the difficult school situation.

The supervisor was not satisfied with the treatment plan developed by the caseworker. The supervisor, who was educated in community social work, believed that the goal of the intervention should be to remedy the dysfunctional family situation through linkage with such resources as health care and housing services. The worker would need to obtain information on the availability of resources in the community, as well as the policies on eligibility for these resources. The economic situation could be improved by helping Mr. Henry to improve his work situation. Also, the supervisor thought that efforts should be made to obtain help from neighbors and the grandmother in relieving Mrs. Smith of some of the day-to-day burdens of family care.

In contrast, the worker thought that the task of finding concrete resources did not require the skills of a professionally trained person, and that this should be delegated to a case aide. Given the long-term nature of the Smith family's problems, the supervisor recommended to the worker that this case should be held open for an indefinite period of time. She assumed that ongoing intervention would obviate child abuse in the future.

The supervisor established work performance standards for the worker, which included environmentally focused case activity. Annual performance evaluations were linked with these performance standards.

Practice in Administration, Community Organization, Policy, and Planning

The difference in orientation to practice between the supervisor and worker was not uncommon in this agency. The hiring policy of this agency was to require training in clinical social work as a prerequisite for direct-service positions. As a result, the goals of the agency were geared to changing service consumers' attitudes and behavior, with less emphasis on environmental change.

The supervisor presented data to the director documenting the problems associated with the hiring of clinically educated workers. The director obtained consent from the board to formulate a new policy, which clarified that the prime goal of the agency would be to change service users', environments. As a result, the agency recruited and hired persons educated in community social work for its direct-service positions.

The administrator also became aware of the difficulties that the direct-service workers had in working with the school system. The schools were not complying with the reporting requirements of the child abuse law. A meeting was established with the school superintendent with preparations made for the development of an affiliation agreement that specified roles and responsibilities of these two organizations with regard to child abuse situations.

Lack of adequate housing for low-income citizens has been a longstanding problem in this community. The Citizens' Committee on Housing was organized as a public advocacy agency to pressure the state to increase subsidized housing for the poor. The community organizer in this agency, upon learning of how lack of housing contributed to child abuse and neglect, assembled child welfare service consumers who were affected by this situation and they agreed to mount a campaign to influence the state.

This precipitated a study by the Community Planning Agency, using statistics provided by the child welfare organization to determine whether the lack of adequate housing was a key factor contributing to child abuse and the placement of children in foster homes. The housing problem would be compounded by a proposed urban renewal program in the downtown area which would further reduce low-income housing.

The community social planner met with the local planning board to express concern at the lack of adequate low-income housing and the negative impact that urban renewal would have on housing for the poor. As a result, the plans for urban renewal were modified to include a proportion of rentals for low-income families.

Another approach taken by the Community Planning Agency to remedy the housing problem was to help facilitate the acceptance of the service users from the child welfare agency into public housing projects. The housing authority was reluctant to accept single-parent families into their projects. The community planner arranged a meeting between the directors of the housing authority and the child welfare agency, which was a first step toward the promulgation of an affiliation agreement between these two agencies.

A complication arose in the efforts to recruit environmentally trained staff. The central office of this state agency had established statewide standards that stressed clinical qualifications for direct service positions in the State Child Protection Agency. These standards were the basis for the state civil service examinations for these positions. Even more significant, the basis for requiring clinically trained staff for child protection work was established in a state statute. The state law on child protection specified that the problems of child abuse required "treatment" of those who were responsible for this abuse. It was also evident that there was little systematic data to evaluate the success of the child abuse law.

When staff in the central office learned of the new hiring policy of the county office, they questioned whether this policy violated state guidelines. The person responsible for state planning in child welfare visited the local agency and learned firsthand of the relevance of environmental interventions in child abuse situations. She subsequently was instrumental in revising the state guidelines for the hiring of child protection workers.

The problem of the state statute still remained. The director of the State Child Protection Agency discussed this situation with the chairman of state legislative committee on human services and convinced her that the statute on child protection needed to be revised. This legislator was aware of this problem through information received from her legislative aide, who, in her job of handling complaints from citizens, had compiled data on this problem. The aide also had the task of helping these citizens to solve their individual problems of finding needed resources. Legislation promulgating new policies to achieve the goals of the child abuse statute was subsequently passed in both houses of the legislature and signed by the governor.

ISSUES

Four issues will be addressed to highlight some of the controversial aspects associated with environmental practice. These issues are: (1) changing people vs. changing environments; (2) environmental practice and professional expertise; (3) environmental practice and the severely disabled; and (4) prevention and environmental practice.

Changing People vs. Changing Environments

The issue of changing people vs. changing environments (Mehr 1980:205) is illustrated in the current emphasis on the ecological perspective in the human services. The ecological approach focuses on the interaction of the person and the environment, with stress on helping the individual to develop the capabilities to adapt to his/her environment (people change), as well as direct modification of the environment (environmental change) (Germain and Gitterman 1980:8; Whittaker et al. 1983:36). The ecological model places much of its emphasis on individual change. Thus, two of Maluccio's (1981:7-8) three components of ecological competence are linked to service consumer capability (service user capacities and skills; service consumer motivation). The model assumes that the person has the capability of "reshaping" systems (Whittaker et al. 1983:33). Germain (1994) also places much responsibility for initiating change on the individual (e.g., change oneself, change one's physical environment, change both environment and self). In contrast, the environmental perspective advocated here claims that individuals have the natural capacity to adapt given a benevolent environment. "Reshaping" systems is the responsibility of professional intervention, and it is inappropriate and overly ambitious to expect service users to achieve this for themselves.

This is illustrated in the case situation. The worker assumed that she could help Mrs. Smith, Mary Jane, and Mr. Henry to cope better with their difficult situation by having them understand better the source of their interpersonal conflicts. She further believed that Mrs. Smith could have the ability to influence the school and deal with the housing situation. In contrast, the supervisor stressed the importance of changing the problematic environments through linkage with formal and informal community resources.

The environmental perspective also assumes that creating positive environments for service consumers require interventions that are *different* from the traditional people-changing technologies. Rothman (1994:17) contrasts traditional classical practice with a "new paradigm" for services to severely vulnerable service users, with the latter focusing on environmental interventions. This new paradigm involves facilitating maintenance of the impaired service consumer in the community; continuous long-term duration of service; meeting multiple needs; linkage to community support resources; practitioner as coordinator of a helping system; and variably sanctioned practitioner authority. Some have suggested that attempts to divide these levels of intervention leads to a false dichotomy (Schwartz 1969). This division is based on the assumption that changing people requires different knowledge and skills than changing policies and structures (Neugeboren 1991:6; Whittaker 1974). Gilbert, Miller, and Specht (1980:37) suggest that environmentally focused practice requires system-oriented interventions which stress *sociopolitical* skills in contrast to the *socioemotional* skills needed for person-change objectives. A similar assumption is made here in the focus on the environment separate from the individual. Another basis for this environmental emphasis is the belief that individuals are often the *victims* of situations (Ryan 1971); therefore the problem lies not in the person, but rather in the external environment (Garvin and Seabury 1984:259-262). The view that social problems are a "private trouble" rather than a "public issue" is evident also in the policies that link homelessness with mental illness rather than with lack of low-cost housing (Hartman 1989:483-484).

In the Smith case, the worker intended to use socioemotional skills to achieve change in family members. The supervisor, in contrast, stressed the need for understanding the policies of the agencies with which the Smith family needed to be linked.

Although change of both the person and the situation might be the ideal goal, time pressures of practice require the establishment of priorities and compels choices as to whether intervention should concentrate on the person *or* the situation (Whitaker et al. 1983:40). Parsimony requires the practitioner to estimate the probability of achieving success in either changing people or chaning situations. Allocation of scarce resources compels the practitioner to make a decision on where change efforts should be directed. Also, claiming to do both at the same time might trivialize either one or the other (Schwartz 1969). The lack of effectiveness of individual change efforts has been documented (Fischer 1973), especially in situations where social and economic deprivation require practical assistance (Frankel 1988:152; Goldberg and Warburton 1979:2) and when dealing with the severely disabled (Rubin 1985). Although evidence comparing the effectiveness of individual vs. situational change interventions is not available, there is some indication that changing policies may be more feasible than changing attitudes

(Mechanic 1974:12). Individual-change strategies may be ineffective because of the unanticipated effects of the environment (Rogers-Warren and Warren 1977).

Environmental Practice and Professional Expertise

A widespread belief among professionals educated in direct practice is that changing service users' attitudes and behavior requires a higher level of knowledge and skill than changing their situations. Consequently, the provision of concrete resources is often relegated to less-trained staff (Harrison 1989:73). Professionalism has therefore become associated with clinical people-changing practice, while linking of service consumers with needed resources is considered less "sophisticated" and deemed "unprofessional" and not "professionally exciting" (Poole 1987:248). Prestige scales that measure social work professional preferences found that social workers had little interest in providing resources to disabled populations (Aviram and Katan 1991). This rejection of service linkage because of the desire for professional status is contradictory to the current practice emphasis on brokerage, and case management (Germain 1994:40).

Rothman (1994:20), in his discussion of standards for community-based "comprehensive enhancement practice," states that proficiency involves across-the-board skills contained in clinical, community, organization, and administrative roles. White (1987:93) suggests that this type of practice requires a breadth of sophistication that exceeds that in the traditional areas of intervention.

In the case, the worker believed that the tasks of linking the service consumer with community resources could be done by a nonprofessional. The supervisor took a different position–she thought it was the responsibility of the professionally trained worker to perform these environmentally focused tasks.

Examination of the tasks involved in environmental manipulation make us aware of the complexity of the required activities associated with this kind of practice (Grinnell and Kyte 1975). For example, helping a severely mentally ill service user obtain housing requires an understanding of the eligibility requirements of the public housing authority (Aviram 1990:73). This includes an awareness of whether the *official* eligibility policies are different from the *operative* regulations and how this might affect the service consumer's access to housing. Linking of the service user with housing might also involve an appreciation of how to influence persons in authority to facilitate the attainment of housing for the service consumer. This task of environmental practice would involve such skills as negotiating for and representing the service user's interests. The competent environmental practitioner needs to understand how bureaucratic structures operate, as well as the basis for coordination of services between agencies (Johnson and Rubin 1983:53; Rothman 1994:20). Community resource coordination will be discussed in Chapters 4 and 5.

In the case, the worker would need to understand the bureaucratic structure of the school system, particularly this system's policy of labeling and underestimating students, in order to adequately negotiate for and represent Mary Jane.

Environmental Practice and the Severely Disabled

The issue of environmental practice for the severely disabled centers on the different needs of the acutely and the severely disabled (Wintersteen 1986:33); the knowledge and skill required to serve these two populations groups; and the interactional effects that chronic disability has on family and the community.

The medicalization of the problem of mental illness illustrates how the medical care system is designed to treat acute illness and not chronic conditions (Aviram 1990:75). The restructuring of community health services for the elderly is related to pressure to medicalize these services, with a consequent reduction in social services (Wood and Estes 1988). Thus, the financial support for acute-care services is proportionately much higher than that for the seriously mentally ill.

The severely disabled, by definition, cannot be "cured." In contrast to interventions for acute problems, service for the severely disabled requires different expectations as to outcomes. This is especially related to expectations as to goals concerned with time and service consumer results. Interventions for the severely disabled require a service strategy that establishes realistic goals within an extended time framework. A model for successful practice with the severely disabled is present in the field of physical rehabilitation. The training of a stroke victim to slowly learn to walk or talk requires perseverance, with the knowledge that within time certain limited objectives are possible. Rothman (1994:21) suggests that success with severely vulnerable service users should be measured not only by "the distance we raise clients, but also the distance we prevent them from falling."

The knowledge and skill required to serve the severely disabled needs to take into account that, by definition, their problems are irreversible and, therefore, service strategies have to accept the ongoing nature of the intervention. Mutual self-help organizations can provide this long-term support (Salem, Seiderman, and Rappaport 1988) needed for "life-style" related illnesses (Shaw and Borkman 1990). This does not mean that gains in service consumer functioning are not possible. It does mean that realistic goals are set, including the limited objective of the prevention or delay of further disability.

Interventions for the severely disabled also have to take into account the impact that disabilities have on family and others in the community, and the consequences this may have for the functioning of the disabled. Given the dependence of the severely disabled on others, professional intervention must recognize the importance of providing support to those who are impacted by the disabled, such as the family. Successful practice with the severely mentally ill involves interventions to improve living environments, as well as the creation and support of service users' social networks (Videka-Sherman 1988). Effective treatment of the severely physically ill requires that medical knowledge be supplemented with a more social approach to deal with such associated problems as social isolation, immobility, social stigmatization, and family disruption (Strauss & Glaser 1975). (See Chapter 9 for an extended discussion of environmental practice for the severely disabled.)

The case situation illustrates the different positions taken by the worker and the supervisor in terms of the chronic versus the acute nature of the problems confronting the Smith family. The worker thought that time-limited intervention was appropriate, in contrast to the supervisor who believed that this case required extended contacts.

Prevention and Environmental Practice

Preventive intervention was pioneered in the public health field in efforts to eradicate communicable diseases. Epidemiological theory focuses on three elements; agent, host, and environment. Traditionally, public health prevention is directed at eliminating agents (e.g., eradicating mosquitoes), strengthening the host (e.g., immunization), and improving the environment (e.g., draining the swamps). The public health definition of prevention (particularly eliminating agents and improving environment) is related to the environmental practice approaches advocated here. Also, the current efforts to combat environmental pollution of air and water points to society's concern with the deleterious effect that the physical environment can have on the well-being of people and the need to engage in preventive efforts to alleviate this threat.

There has been hope that this preventive public health framework can be transferred to the field of the human services (Caplan 1964; Wittman 1978). However, there is little evidence that early interventions will prevent mental health problems from occurring in the future (Gilbert 1982; Mechanic 1980). But if we assume that environmental factors are the principle cause of various social problems, then interventions which utilize this knowledge can be expected to prevent future occurrence of these problems. (See Chapter 6 for a discussion of the relation of social support to prevention.) In the case, prevention of further child abuse was assumed possible through intervention that changed either the person or the environment.

DEFINITION OF ENVIRONMENTAL PRACTICE

Environment as Context vs. Target for Practice

It is useful to differentiate the environment as the context from the environment as a target for practice. This distinction is noted in the CSWE accrediting standards for social work education (Curriculum Policy Statement 1992:M5.4.3). The effect of environmental contexts on practice models will be discussed throughout this book in addition to interventions to modify environments.

The *context* relates to how the environment can *constrain or facilitate* professional activities (Neugeboren 1991:xii-xiii), affecting consumer benefit. The CSWE policy for Human Behavior and Social Environment curricula requires information on how "systems promote and deter people in the maintenance or attainment of optimal health and well being" (Curriculum Policy Statement 1992:M6.9) (i.e., the context of practice). For example, agency goals and structures can facilitate or constrain professional practice. Thus, the agency goal of rehabilitation will constrain a direct-service worker from working towards the goal of changing environments, while it will facilitate efforts to change service user attitudes and behavior. The context of agency structure can also constrain or facilitate practice. For example, a clear role structure that defines behavior expectations for staff can facilitate practice, whereas an ambiguous one will constrain performance by producing role strain and conflict. Knowledge of how the environment influences practice facilitates successful *use of structure*, enabling navigation of the system by minimizing constraints and maximizing opportunities for action.

An understanding of how the environment constrains and facilitates practice is necessary on both on the macro and micro intervention levels. In the above example, the deficient role structure can be overcome by the direct practitioner by working with the supervisor in clarifying the particular worker's job expectations. The task of skillful use of structure falls particularly within the province of the direct-service practitioner. On the macro level, the problem of a defective role structure requires the administrator to take this into account in the management of staff performance-evaluation systems.

Another option would be for the administrator to change the policy on staff roles. This establishes the environment as the *target* of practice. The environment as the target for practice emphasizes efforts to *change* environments. The focus here is change of policies and structures by macro environmental practitioners: administrators, planners, and policymakers. The above discussion focused on how the *organization* is the target of practice. The *community* as the target for intervention has regained the attention of social policy analysts and planners (Thurz and Vigilante 1978). "Social work's objective is to strengthen the community's capacities to solve problems through development of groups and organizations, community education, community systems of governance and control over systems of social care." (Specht and Courtney 1994:27). Deinstitutionalization has created pressure to reclaim the community as a strategy for integration of the severely disabled (Sullivan 1992). (Interventions to strengthen informal community care systems are discussed in Chapters 6 and 7 on social support.)

The issue of whether society supports professional efforts to change communities has been raised (Saxton 1991:314). Are there *jobs* for community change agents? Although in the poverty programs in the 1960's there was funding for community organization efforts to target communities for change, this support has since diminished. However, a function of community social planning is to make communities more functional in meeting human needs. Whether community planners take on this mission or not, it is part of their legitimate role and function. Responsibility for building "healthy" communities falls on other professionals as well, such as administrators of community agencies, whose role it is to work with others to improve the community resource system so that their service users will receive the resources they need. Therefore, the intervention knowledge and skill to change communities is required by community planners, as well as by agency administrators and staff.

Therefore, the distinction between the environment as the context and as the target for practice is linked with the difference between using and changing structure, which will be discussed next.

Using vs. Changing Environments

Environmental practice can be directed toward better use of and/ or changing existing service delivery environments. Effective *use* of environments requires an understanding of existing policies in order to maximize service consumer benefit. Therefore, enhancing the use of environments means improving service access. This includes a focus on "environmental resource development," as well as mobilizing and managing service consumers living, learning, and working environments (Anthony and Lieberman 1986; Vosler 1990). Facilitating usage of existing services is associated with the role of the direct-practice worker. Intervention to *change* environments involves modification of policies and structures by administrators, community organizers, planners, and policymakers in order to create more functional service delivery systems. This definition of environmental practice is similar to that of "social care" formulated by Robert Morris (1977). Social care is

> The creation and management of social environments . . . specific tasks include (1) identifying which persons need care . . . would deemphasize belief that their needs can be best met by intervention designed to cure. (2) The profession (social work) would develop social policy and act as an advocate for persons who are the victims of this complex technological society. (Morris 1977:357).

We see in the case situation that intervention could have been directed at the living, learning, and working environments of the Smith family. The worker could have modified the living situation by exploring the availability of more-adequate housing, possibly in low-income, subsidized apartments. The situation at Mary Jane's school required intervention to deal with possible labeling of Mary Jane as "slow," resulting in low expectations of her school performance. Mr. Henry's working situation could be the target of intervention in the effort to explore opportunities for vocational training.

Functional Community

Environmental intervention is directed at agency and community aspects of service delivery. Focus is on the service user's *functional community*: "those institutional arrangements and socioeconomic conditions in which service consumers transact their daily lives and acquire or fail to acquire the resources needed to maintain their health and welfare" (Austin and Patti 1984:10-12). This functional community, which includes such services as employment, education, housing, and recreation, may have deficits that impact on service users and need to be circumvented or may have untapped resources that need to be mobilized for service consumer benefit. (See Chapters 4 and 5 on community resource coordination.)

The importance of employment as resource received a renewed recognition in the welfare reform of the Reagan administration (Family Support Act of 1988) and in the Clinton welfare plans, as well as in the Contract for America formulated in 1995 by congressional Republicans. The roles of direct-service workers, managers, staff developers, policy analysts, advocates, and social researchers in implementing work strategies for welfare mothers has been delineated (Hagen 1992:11-13). However, work as a viable strategy for eliminating poverty has been questioned, given the economic vulnerability of the single parent. Thus, although Swedish single mothers have high levels of work force participation, they still require financial assistance to supplement their wages (Rosenthal 1994).

The environmental factor in the PIE Scale classifies "functional community" by utilizing Warren's community systems format of economic; education; legal; health, safety and welfare; and voluntary association systems (Warren 1963). A sixth community system, "affectional support system," referring to service user's social support system, was added (Karls and Wandrei 1994:23-34).

Family Access to Basic Resources (FABR) (Vosler 1990) is an assessment tool used by direct-service workers to map specific family economic stresses from lack of access to adequate and stable basic resources. Documentation of a family's lack of access can be used as a base for advocacy, public education, lobbying, and multilevel systems change.

The "functional community" of the Smith family included the systems that could provide the resources they needed to function, such as employment, housing, and health care.

Organizational Environment

The social agency is also a potential target for environmental interventions (Garvin and Seabury 1984:162-189). "The policies and practices of an agency, its leadership, its socioemotional climate and culture are likely to have an influence on service consumer's attitudes toward and involvement in the service experience" (Austin and Patti 1984:12). Environmental practice is directed at influencing this agency environment to maximize the opportunities and minimize the constraints of organizational contextual factors (Neugeboren 1991). (See Chapter 8 on organizational environments.)

The organizational environment of the school which seemed to underestimate Mary Jane could have been a target of intervention for the worker, addressing the possible existence of school policies that encouraged labeling of students.

Vulnerable Populations

As indicated earlier, intervention in the environment has particular relevance for groups such as the mentally ill, developmentally disabled, alcoholics (Cocozzelli and Hudson 1989:540-545), the physically disabled, and frail elderly (Commission on Chronic Illness 1956), who cannot be expected to be "cured" of their problems, but nevertheless could benefit from more benevolent environments (DeWeaver 1983:436; Mechanic 1986; Segal and Baumohl 1980). Rothman (1994:3) states that severely vulnerable populations have expanded in numbers, requiring new-service delivery models consisting of protracted and multifaceted services extending over a lifetime.

A basic assumption underlying environmental practice is that service users are motivated and have the competence to constructively use social opportunities when they are appropriate for their needs. We therefore view service consumers in terms of their *strengths* and are careful not to underestimate their capacities by overemphasis on pathology. A comparison of social worker and service user perceptions indicates that the former underestimate the service consumer's strengths (Maluccio 1981). The strength perspective is advocated for persons released from mental institutions (Sullivan 1992). This approach can have a supportive effect (Ballew & Mink 1986; Lamb 1980; Weick et al. 1989). In general, environmental practice occurs in a *high-expectation milieu* to avoid stress on weaknesses and creating dependency (Wood and Middleman 1989). An example of the value of a high-expectation environment is the Lodge experiment in which schizophrenics successfully operated a house cleaning business (Fairweather 1969). The reader will note in this book the absence of the term "client," which implies dependency. Terms such as consumer, customer, or user, are employed instead (Specht and Courtney 1994:154), to signify that the person served has the ability to evaluate services which he/she can accept or refuse. In one poverty program, the term "resident" was used to connote that the service consumer was entitled to service as a member of a community (Neugeboren 1970b). In Puerto Rico, the term "beneficiary" is used to refer to consumers of public welfare services, also implying their entitlement to this aid.

Environmental Manipulation

The emphasis of practice on changing environments is similar to the *environmental manipulation* stressed in the early years of the social work profession. It is concerned not only with physical environments, but also social ecology–the study of human milieus (Moos 1974a:22-30). Quality-of-life scales used to assess environmental impact in long-term care include such measurements as: service user's perception of control, freedom, choice, and autonomy permitted by the environment; structure, rules, and expected behavior imposed by the environment; and relationships between individuals and caregivers in the environment (Kane and Kane 1984). Environmental practice uses data on service consumers' quality of life to design interventions that can constructively modify environments.

Environmental manipulation combats the problem of social isolation, which is a critical factor contributing to and compounding the problems associated with physical and social disability (Garbarino 1980:7). Therefore, intrinsic to the creation of functional environments for the disabled is the promotion of supportive social networks that are required in modern society but are no longer adequately provided by the extended family (Morris 1977:354-355). (See Chapters 6 and 7 on social support.) The isolation of the Smith family could have been remedied by creating support links between the family and the grandmother and neighbors.

SUMMARY

This chapter has introduced the area of environmental practice by contrasting this approach to the more traditional form of service that is concerned with changing service users' attitudes and behavior. Four issues were considered: the alternative service strategies of changing people vs. changing their environments; whether environmental practice requires professional expertise; the relevance of this type of practice for the acutely or severely disabled; and whether environmental practice could have prevention as a goal.

Environmental practice was defined by contrasting the concept of environment as a context or as a target of practice. Two types of intervention targets—using vs. changing the environment—were addressed as was the relationship of environmental practice with the functional community, organizational environments, vulnerable populations, and environmental manipulation.

STUDY QUESTIONS

1. Discuss the need for environmental practice in view of the history of this practice and previous efforts to develop this type of intervention.

2. Present the pros and cons of changing individuals vs. changing their environments, referring to the case on child abuse.

3. Examine the issue of professional expertise and status in relationship to engaging in practice with vulnerable populations.

4. Address the pros and cons of doing preventive interventions as part of environmental practice.

5. Discuss how the environment can be viewed as the context of practice. Cite examples of how the context can constrain and facilitate practice.

6. Using the case, illustrate how the concept of using vs. changing environment is relevant.

7. Examine a personal experience that illustrates how the organizational environment helped and/or hindered your work.

8. Debate how environmental manipulation can be used to assist vulnerable populations.

Chapter 2

FRAMEWORK FOR AN ENVIRONMENTAL PRACTICE TECHNOLOGY

Framework for an Environmental Practice Technology

I.   An Environmental Practice Technology
II.   Practice Models in the Human Services
     A. Maximizing Environmental Opportunities
III.   Organizational Context: Opportunities and Constraints
        on Practice
IV.   Practice Levels
     A. Micro Level: Changing Service User Situations
     B. Macro Level: Changing Policies
V.   Practice Arenas
     A. Organizational Arenas
        1. Micro Level: Case Work
        2. Macro Level: Administration
           a. Formulation of Direct-Service Agency Goals
           b. Design of Organizational Structures
           c. Program Implementation
     B. Community Arena
        1. Micro Level: Social Advocacy
        2. Macro Level: Community Planning
           a. Community Needs Assessment
           b. Facilitation of Inter-Agency Coordination
           c. Monitoring and Feedback
     C. Societal Arena: Social Policy Formulating Agencies
        1. Micro Level: Legislative Aide
        2. Macro Level: Social Policy Analyst
VI.   Policy Analysis Framework
     A. Changes in Substantive Goals
     B. Changes in Strategies for Achieving Goals
        1. Internal Change
           a. Organizational Assessment
        2. External Change

VII. Integration of Micro and Macro Environmental Practice
    A. Common and Specific Knowledge and Skill
    B. Cooperation vs. Conflict Between Micro
       and Macro Practitioners
    C. Interdependency Between Micro and Macro Practice
VIII. Practice Skills
    A. Practice Skills in Direct Practice, Administration,
       Planning, and Policy
IX. Summary
X. Study Questions

AN ENVIRONMENTAL PRACTICE TECHNOLOGY

This chapter presents a conceptual framework which will be used to guide the subsequent explication of an environmental practice technology. Hasenfeld (1983) defines a human service technology as "a set of institutionalized procedures aimed at changing the physical, psychological, social or cultural attributes of people in order to transform them from a given status to a new prescribed status" (p. 111). An environmental practice technology will need to focus on the "social" aspects of service user situations. It will target environmental factors that need to be changed in order to move the service consumer to a new, more functional status. It is similar to people-processing technologies designed to "confer on people a particular social label, social position, or status that will, in turn, produce a predetermined response from significant social groups or organizations" (Hasenfeld 1972:135). But it has a more positive goal of enhancing social functioning, in contrast to people processing, which has the objective of classification and referral. Since environmental interventions by definition are directed outward, practitioner activities are heavily involved in interorganizational exchanges. The model of environmental technology presented here is based on the integration of existing practice roles. It is linked to micro and macro roles in the three intervention arenas: direct service, community planning and social advocacy, and social policy agencies.

This chapter begins by reviewing several practice frameworks previously developed in the human services, indicating how these relate to the one used in this book. The organizational contexts creating opportunities and constraints on practice that have been part of previous frameworks will be integrated into the framework used here through the differentiation in practice between micro and macro levels and the three practice arenas. The relationships between micro and macro environmental interventions will be analyzed to indicate how practice on these two levels could be integrated. This chapter concludes with a brief review of six practice skills common to both micro and macro environmental practice. The case presented in Chapter 1 will be used to illustrate how the framework applies to practice.

PRACTICE MODELS IN THE HUMAN SERVICES

Practice models in the human services have varied over time. The field started with casework, followed by group work, community organization, administration, planning and policy, and research. In recent years, generic or integrated models for practice have been developed. However, the generic models have been seen as "new wine in old bottles," in that they emphasize primarily intervention on the micro level (Schwartz 1977; Neugeboren 1986).

A variety of macro practice models are relevant for environmental practice. These frameworks specify practitioner roles, functions, skills, and contexts. Perlman and Gurin (1972) classified community organization and social planning according to three organizational contexts: voluntary associations; service agencies; and planning organizations. Rothman (1979) also used the practice function in defining community organization according to locality development, social action, and social planning. Patti (1983) specifies the principal tasks in administration practice according to a developmental context that includes three stages: design, implementation, and stabilization. Relevant activities include: planning program development; acquiring financial resources and support; designing organizational structures; developing and maintaining staff capability; and assessing and changing agency programs. Mintzberg (1973) specifies three major roles in administration as interpersonal, informational, and decisional. Austin (1986) combines the Rothman and Mintzberg models to propose a model for integrating community organization and administration practice. These different models specify skills that are needed to perform different roles and functions.

A practice framework developed by Middleman and Goldberg (1974) aims to adjust the environment to the needs of the individual a goal similar to that of the model presented here. It is based on two dimensions: locus of concern and person(s) engaged. Efforts can be directed at dealing with the problems of individuals or groups of persons with similar difficulties by engaging not only the client but also nonclients (e.g., neighbors, politicians, other professionals).

Weissman, Epstein, and Savage (1983) also propose a model which stresses nontraditional practice roles and functions, which they state are the neglected aspects of clinical practice. Some of these are: diagnostician, expeditor, case manager, colleague, advocate, program developer, organizational reformer, supervisor, practice researcher, and employee.

Maximizing Environmental Opportunities

The PIE mentioned in Chapter 1 provides a detailed codification of environmental problems that could be used as a guide for environmental interventions. Its focus is on the absence of community resources in five community systems: economic; education; judicial; health and welfare; and voluntary associations. Although the PIE scale provides a useful system for codification of environmental barriers to service user social functioning, it emphasizes the *absence* of community resources. For example, under the category of employment, subcategories: unemployment (employment not available); underemployment (adequate employment is not available) and inappropriate employment (lack of socially and legally acceptable employment) (Karls and Wandrei 1994). The focus on environmental barriers precludes searching for environmental opportunities. For example, the problem of underemployment might be remedied by the professional seeking ways to help the service consumer find a job more suitable for his/her abilities and skills.

The PIE scale does have some potential for constructive interventions in the area of discrimination, which is included as an environmental barrier in the affectional support system. Successful professional action is possible in this area since antidiscrimination laws provide the sanction that the professional can use to overcome this environmental barrier.

The definition of environmental practice used here emphasizes opportunities as well as constraints, with special attention given to how professional intervention can overcome the environmental constraints while maximizing opportunities.

ORGANIZATIONAL CONTEXT: OPPORTUNITIES AND CONSTRAINTS ON PRACTICE

The influence of organizational context on community organization practice was initially conceptualized by Zald (1965:4). The conceptual framework proposed here also draws on the assumption made in the Perlman (1972), Rothman (1979), and Patti (1983) models that the context in which the practice occurs has a significant influence on its content. Thus, situational factors need to be taken into account for practice to be effective.

The auspices under which an agency operates can constrain or facilitate interventions. Public agencies have different service-delivery patterns than those under voluntary nonprofit sponsorship (Neugeboren 1970a). The potential for use of conflict strategies required for social advocacy will depend on whether a given agency provides the sanction for this type of intervention (Perlman and Gurin 1972:76). Thus, organizations that have advocacy as a prime goal (e.g., citizen's committees advocating for the mentally ill, children, or developmentally disabled, public advocates, etc.) derive opportunities from the sanction to do service user advocacy. In contrast, direct-service and planning agencies, which do not have this sanction, are constrained from engaging in the conflict strategies required to do advocacy. Lack of appreciation of contextual constraints can have negative personal consequences for practitioners who attempt to perform service consumer advocacy without organizational support (Westman 1991). Weissman, Epstein, and Savage (1983) discuss the "hazards of advocacy," including potential job loss. Patti (1974) cites other undesirable consequences of internal advocacy, including embarrassment with friends and family, income loss, forced geographic mobility, and the burden of explaining negative job references.

Middleman and Goldberg (1974) discuss an aspect of organizational context that they call "metawork": all those activities that are not performed directly with service users (e.g., supervisory conferences, staff meetings, paperwork, etc.). Although they characterize metawork as generally facilitating the actual service work (p. 154), they also recognize that the large amount of time spent in processing activities can detract from the work performed directly with service consumers. Thus, metawork is both a constraint and a facilitator of practice. The environmental practitioner should understand these contextual opportunities and constraints in order to maximize the former and minimize the latter.

The conceptual model proposed here differs from traditional frameworks. For example, rather than separating practice into community organization and administration, it presumes that the skills and tasks needed in these areas are similar, even though their application is different in accordance with the opportunities and constraints of the practice contexts. For example, the manner in which direct-service agency administrators use leadership, negotiating, and representing skills to gain support and legitimation from external constituencies differs from that of the community organizer who lacks the legitimate power available to the manager. It also proposes that the application of these skills that are generic to both macro and micro level practice will vary somewhat depending on whether the target is an individual or a system.

As indicated, environmental intervention occurs on different levels and in different arenas, all of which presents different opportunities and constraints for practice. There are micro and macro levels of practice (Mehr 1980:2). Micro practice refers to direct services, for both individuals and groups. Macro intervention includes administration, social planning, and social policy formulation. The three contextual arenas of practice are: organization, community, and societal (Meyer et al. 1967). Environmental practice can be directed at changing situations for service users on an individual or group basis and/or changing policies and structures to create more functional environments for groups of service consumers.

The significance of context stems from the varying authority, legitimacy, and sanctions supporting or constraining practitioner's actions at each level and in each arena. Practitioner roles (e.g., direct-service provider, administrator, planner, policy analyst) have imbedded in them socially sanctioned limits that require the practitioner to act in fairly circumscribed ways. This concept contrasts with other practice models (e.g., Middleman and Goldberg 1974; Weissman et al. 1983) that propose that certain activities can be performed by all practitioners, regardless of their official roles and functions.

Although this framework for environmental practice separates micro and macro practice on the basis of their different targets of intervention, the linkage between these levels of practice needs to be considered. The *interdependencies* between micro and macro practice require ongoing communication between these levels of intervention, a factor that will be addressed later in the chapter in the section on *integration* of micro and macro practice.

The following chart summarizes this framework for environmental practice:

Framework for Environmental Practice

ARENA   LEVEL

	Micro Changing individual situations	Macro Changing policies
Organization Direct-Service Agency	Case worker Help service user to negotiate systems to obtain resources	Administrator Formulate goals; design and implement programs
Community Community Planning and Social Advocacy Agencies	Community Organizer Advocacy with service consumer groups	Planner Need assessment; agency coordination; allocation of resources
Society Policy Formulating Agencies– Legislature	Legislative aide Link between citizens and legislators	Policy Analyst Change goals and strategies to achieve goals

PRACTICE SKILLS

Decision Making Negotiating	Monitoring Representing	Leadership Staffing

The following discussion of the framework begins with micro and macro practice levels, then the three contextual arenas, and lastly the generic practice skills. Examples from environmental theory and research are cited to illustrate the relevance of these concepts to different practice situations.

PRACTICE LEVELS

Micro Level: Changing Service User Situations

Case-level interventions involve representing service consumers (individuals, as well as groups) in the various systems from which they have to obtain assistance. Direct practitioners work with individual service users to help them change their situations. Community organizers work with groups of service consumers representing their interests as service users. Whether it is a housing authority that discriminates against single-parent families or a public assistance agency that unlawfully restricts its services, practice on the micro level is focused on influencing the application of policies that impede individual service consumer benefit. Case management (Rapp and Chamberlain 1985) and discharge planning are examples of micro level interventions. Case managers, armed with an understanding of how organizational environments can be functional or dysfunctional for service users, can use this information in referring service consumers to those programs that have beneficial milieus. For example, research in social ecology indicates that smaller organizations place more emphasis on relationships with service users and deemphasize control (Moos 1974a:331). Whittaker (1974) includes "indirect intervention on behalf of clients" as part of "social treatment," observing that it is an attempt to put the "social" back into social work practice (167). Effective practice depends on the worker having knowledge of the various social systems in which the service consumer participates (e.g., family, peer group, organization, and community), as well on how to influence (e.g., bases of power) these systems (168-172).

In the case of the Smith familly discussed earlier, the role of the direct-service worker as defined by the supervisor is consistent with the above definition of micro environmental practice. This role placed emphasis on linking of service user with community resources.

Macro Level: Changing Policies

Macro environmental practice is that area of professional intervention that involves policy, planning, and administration of social care programs. In contrast with the micro level, where emphasis is on changing situations for individual service consumers, the macro level is concerned with changing policies and structures.

On the *policy formulation* arena, intervention modifies and/or creates legislation that shapes the environment so as to enable the provision of the needed resources. For example, housing policies might be developed that enable deinstitutionalized persons to live in the least restrictive environment. Health financing policies which are institutionally biased would be changed to enable the disabled to remain in the community. Government funding might be allocated for community support services to facilitate self-help programs and other supportive interventions to help maintain the severely disabled in the community. U.S. Social Security policies that provide disincentives for the disabled to become independent would be modified (Aviram 1990:78). The policy formulation role was illustrated in the Smith case where the central office staff proposed an expansion of the child protection statute to include an environmental purpose.

Macro level practice in the community is concerned with *community planning* and *social advocacy*. Community planning is directed at more effective allocation of existing funds to ensure that the disabled are given their share of service resources. Planning interventions would also be concerned with better coordination of existing services, since the disabled require a multiplicity of services. Intrinsic to planning is program evaluation directed at environmental assessment (Knight 1980). Social advocacy is performed by community organizers who represent groups of service users through citizen advocacy agencies. Community organizers also engage in social advocacy in their work with self-help groups. Social advocates whose engagement with service consumers provide them with information about community needs and concerns, are uniquely positioned to represent service users' interests. This information can be used by professionals to evaluate organizational environments, such as their climates and behavior settings (see Chapter 8). Community organizers can then provide information to administrators, planners, and policy analysts on program effects as perceived by service consumers.

The community planning role was illustrated in the Smith case where the central office staff developed new guidelines for the recruitment and selection of staff at the Child Protection Agency. The social advocacy function was illustrated by the work done by the Citizens' Committee on Housing.

In the *direct-service agency*, macro level intervention is directed at modifying existing policies, structures, and technologies to enable more effective provision of social care services. Rothman's

(1994:266-268) study of case management practice with the severely disabled found six areas of organizational problems that would require administrative action: work overload; deficiencies in field operations; lack of organizational coherence and stability; inadequate staff development and support; inadequate service consumer centeredness; and lack of resources. In the area of staff development, particular attention needs to be given to the kinds of knowledge and skill required to serve the severely disabled, especially in terms of the expectations for change and "cure."

In the Smith case, the administrator changed agency hiring policies to recruit environmentally trained practitioners. The administrator also needed to recruit supervisory and administrative staff who had the knowledge and skill to implement an environmentally oriented child protection program.

PRACTICE ARENAS

Micro and macro environmental practice occurs in three arenas: direct-service organizations (mental health and child welfare services); social advocacy agencies (e.g., citizen committees for the mentally ill) and community planning organizations (e.g., United Way, city and county planning and allocating agencies); and social policy formulating agencies (e.g., legislative bodies, national and state central offices of human service programs). The following sections discuss micro and macro practice in these three arenas.

Organizational Arenas

Micro Level: Case Work

Micro interventions in direct-service agencies modify situations for individual service users. Work with individual service consumers is performed by direct service practitioners.

Environmentally focused direct-service interventions apply individual situational analysis (Neugeboren 1991:285-286) to assess the different policy and program barriers that hinder the attainment of needed resources. Micro environmental practice on the organizational level helps service consumers navigate and negotiate these systemic barriers. In the case, for example, the supervisor did a situational analysis of the Smith family and concluded that intervention was needed to link this family with such community resources as housing and health care. Some of the environmental interventions used in direct-service include resource provision, least restrictive environment, normalization, opening opportunity structures, people processing, case management and discharge planning, and social support (Neugeboren 1991:274-285).

Resource provision makes available concrete resources such as medical care, money, housing, and jobs (Ewalt and Honeyfield 1981; Gilbert and Specht 1974; Torczyner and Pare 1979). The practitioner assists the consumer in overcoming the institutional barriers to "access to and use of social utilities" (Siporin 1975:140). It requires working with such agencies as social security, public welfare, and public schools with an understanding of their policies, regulations, procedures and forms. In the case, the worker would need to understand the policies of the school before intervening to change the situation in which Mary Jane was labeled as "slow," resulting in unrealistically low expectations of her.

Environmental practice in direct-service agencies is sensitive to the importance of the *least restrictive environment* for disabled persons (Lamb and Peele 1984:799). This is related to the legal principle of "least restrictive alternative," which states that government should use methods that curtail individual freedom to a minimal extent and should resist community pressure for social control (Chambers 1975:25, 29). Direct-service interventions should take into account the degree of environmental restrictiveness of the various agencies that they are considering for possible referral of their service users. The worker in the case situation has to assess the restrictiveness of the school situation (e.g., placement of Mary Jane in a special class for slow learners) in order to determine whether transfer to a less-restrictive environment might be indicated.

Environmental practitioners in direct-service agencies also apply the principle of *normalization* in their interventions (Cnaan et al. 1988). Normalization has been defined by Wolfensberger (1972:28) as the use of culturally normative means for achieving personal behaviors that approximate that which is culturally normal. Because normalization attempts to achieve "normative" behavior, it requires an understanding of the phenomena of social deviancy, including the potential reinforcement of deviancy by the community's biased expectations (e.g., stigma). Direct practice technologies use normalization concepts to " undo the stigma" (Goffman 1963; Lowenberg 1981). This principle was applied in the Lodge experiment (Fairweather 1969), where schizophrenics were set up in a normalized, high-expectation housecleaning business. Direct-service environmental practice uses the principles of normalization to assess the adequacy of efforts to assist their service consumers to achieve levels of behavior that approximate normalized standards.

In the case situation, Mary Jane was labeled as "slow," even though she tested as having normal intelligence. An intervention objective would be to "undo the stigma" by influencing the teacher and persons of authority that Mary Jane had normal ability and that the expectations of her should therefore be the same as for the other children.

Environmental practice on the direct-service level also deals with *opportunity structures opening,* an approach that was emphasized in the poverty programs of the 1960s. The concept is derived from sociological theory on juvenile delinquency that attributes deviant behavior to a "disjuncture between cultural goals and socially structured opportunity" (Cloward 1959). When legitimate means for goal achievement are unavailable, individuals will turn to illegitimate means. Members of the lower socioeconomic classes have a restricted opportunity structure (i.e., lack connections) in such areas as jobs and education. Micro practice intervenes in such opportunity structures as education, housing, and employment to facilitate successful use of these opportunities (Neugeboren 1970b).

The worker in the case could intervene in the opportunity structures of housing and employment. Connections could be made with subsidized housing programs to enable the Smith family to move to more adequate quarters. Mr. Henry, might be assisted in locating a training program to upgrade his skills and enhance his opportunities for future employment.

People processing (Hasenfeld 1972) is a direct-service environmental intervention that focuses on facilitating status change. A person's public identity (status) can influence societal and self-reaction if the social position is an inferior or stigmatized one (e.g., former mental patient, ex-convict). The concept of the patient "career" (Goffman 1961:125-169), with the mental patient moving from prepatient to inpatient to ex-patient status, captures the way in which human service agencies can affect the public status of persons served. Social labeling can limit social opportunities through stigmatization. The object of the environmental practitioner is destigmitization and delabeling by obviating the placement of the person in an inferior status (e.g., sick role) leading to lower social expectations in such situations as job or school. The environmental worker needs to counteract the tendency to err on the side of classifying individuals as sick in order to minimize risk to themselves if they make an incorrect diagnosis (Scheff 1968:105).

In the case, Mary Jane was labeled as "slow" and placed in a special class, even though she tested at a normal level of intelligence. Intervention to "destigmatize" Mary Jane requires that the worker influence the school to transfer Mary Jane back to a regular class and provide her with any specialized help she requires to perform her schoolwork.

Discharge planning and *case management* are other examples of environmentaly focused direct-practice interventions. The aspect of this practice that relates to environmental factors is the service linkage function essential to case management and discharge planning (Austin 1983; Kane 1980). The two are interrelated through the continuum from discharge from institutional care to case management in the community to insure adequate postinstitutional adjustment. Both functions require skills in interagency service coordination (see Chapters 4 and 5 on community resource coordination). The worker in the Smith case needed to do case management to link the family with such community resources as health and employment-training services.

Environmental practice in direct service also involves *resource coordination* (see Chapter 4) between agencies to accomplish service integration for service users who require resources from different organizations. Resource coordination is related to the "community social work" that has been developed in Great Britain, where direct services involve "networked based helping by families, neighbors, coworkers, and other members of the community" (Harrison and Hoshino

1985:215). In contrast to a case-by-case approach, it employs a "collective redefinition of problems and social work tasks and methods" (Harrison 1987:395).

Intrinsic to environmental practice in the community is the provision of *social support* (see Chapters 6 and 7). Studies of help-seeking behavior reveals that 95 percent of help-seeking interactions occur with such informal caregivers as family, physicians, clergy, managers on the job, hairdressers, bartenders, and pharmacists (Gottlieb 1985:295). Informal networking enables the linking of people through social ties to facilitate the generation and exchange of resources, and provides the basis for the "most organized and visible alternative to professional help–mutual aid and support groups" (Gottlieb 1985:296). Network analysis allows the mapping of primary networks. Some of the dimensions used for social mapping are: (1) structural: size, composition, degree of connectiveness, and geographic dispersion; and (2) procedural: type of helping exchanges, degree of reciprocity; and levels of relational intimacy. Five types of support are: (1) socializing and companionship; (2) emotional support; (3) advice and guidance; (4) tangible aid; and (5) esteem support. These dimensions can be used to assess the social world of the service user, leading to strategies for changing networks to enhance their utility. This framework has been applied to clinical casework and protective services (Gottlieb 1985).

Community support strategies have also been applied to mental health, medical and work contexts, and informal care among the elderly (Gottlieb 1983:145-203; Biegel, Shore, and Gordon 1984; Kaye 1985; Crotty and Kulys 1985; Stein 1979). As indicated above with regard to normalization, intervention in community networks also has relevance for the alleviation of social isolation.

In the case situation, the worker needed to assess the community network of the Smith family to determine where support might be possible. This might include help from Mary Jane's father and grandmother, as well as aid from neighbors and friends.

Other environmental interventions in direct service include habilitation (Wiegerink and Pelosi 1979) and social ecology (Moos 1974a) (see Chapter 8). These environmental approaches as well as those discussed above have received more detailed treatment under the classification of social care technologies (Neugeboren 1991:269-286).

Macro Level: Administration

Macro interventions in direct-service organizations are performed by the administrator who must fulfill three functions: (1) formulation of environmentally oriented agency goals; (2) design of organizational structures relevant for these goals; and (3) directing staff in the implementation of these goals.

Formulation of Direct-service Agency Goals. Formulation of environmentally relevant goals requires that the direct-service agency administrator obtain support and sanction from funding authorities, governing boards, and staff to establish direct-service programs to create benevolent environments for service consumers. "Institutional leadership" (Selznick 1957) is required to convince these groups to accept a major shift from the traditional rehabilitation goals. The establishment of environmentally centered official goals is required in order to legitimate the reallocation of resources and to overcome the resistance of those who have commitments to the traditional people-change service modalities (Neugeboren 1991:182-188). In the Smith case, the director of the agency obtained support from the board to formulate a new policy that shifted the goals of the agency from rehabilitation of individual service users to changing dysfunctional environments.

The shift to environmentally oriented agency goals should be based on an assessment of existing policies that have been found to hinder service consumer benefit. Policies that promote interagency cooperation through the development of affiliation agreements are necessary for effective programming for the disabled, who require a multiplicity of services that cannot be provided by any single agency. In the Smith case, the director changed the hiring policy of the agency after determining that the existing policy of recruiting clinically educated staff was inappropriate for agency goals.

The formulation of environmentally oriented organizational goals utilizes conceptual and empirical tools from the field of social ecology (Moos 1974a) to create more functional agency environments (see Chapter 8). This framework is used to specify what aspects of the agency environment require modification, whether they be the architectural aspects, the behavior expectations of service consumers, and/or the organizational climate.

The Multiphasic Environmental Assessment Procedure (MEAP) (Moos and Lemke 1984) systematically measures some of these social and physical dimensions of organizations and has been used in sheltered care settings such as nursing homes, residential care facilities, and congregate apartments. This instrument has been widely tested with norms developed from findings in 244 facilities. The results of the data obtained through the use of MEAP are used by administrators to clarify goals, to suggest facility modification, and to monitor the results of program change (Moos and Lemke 1984:73).

In the case situation, the director could assess the climate of the agency by determining staff expectations for service users. If expectations were found to be low, then policy changes could be made to rectify this.

The formulation of environmentally oriented organizational goals of direct-service agencies also includes the creation of "normalized" environments for service consumers (Wolfensberger 1972). Program Analysis of Service Systems (PASS) (Wolfensberger and Glenn 1975) can be used to evaluate the extent to which a service meets the criteria and ideals of the principle of normalization. The goal of normalization is integration of socially deviant service users, and PASS is a systematic procedure for assessing how successfully an organization or community is pursuing that goal. Some of the categories used in the assessment are: (1) physical integration; (2) social integration; (3) age appropriate interpretations and structures; (4) culture appropriate interpretations and structures; (5) developmental growth orientation; and (6) quality of setting. The administrator of thr child welfare agency in the Smith case could use PASS to assess the extent to which the agency meets normalization standards (e.g., the degree that the families supervised by this agency are integrated into the community).

Design of Organizational Structures. Achievement of environmentally oriented agency goals requires the design of structures appropriate to the accomplishment of these objectives. Five types of structures are involved: role, authority, communication, reward, and interorganizational relations (Indik and Berrien 1968:7-8).

The *role* structure specifies staff job expectations at the direct service and supervisory levels. Environmental programs require the design of staff roles for such tasks as seeking and obtaining resources for service consumers. Community resource coordination roles on the micro and macro levels are central to environmental practice (see Chapters 5 and 6). In the Smith case, the disagreement between the worker and supervisor could have been avoided if the agency had defined the direct service role in terms of linking service users with resources.

Communication structures specify what and to whom information is directed. Since environmental practice requires integration of direct-service and administrative efforts, formalized systems for intraorganizational communication to achieve coordination must be designed. In the Smith case, communication from the service-delivery level to administration was useful in informing the administration of the dysfunctional hiring policy. Interorganizational coordination requires the design of channels of communication between agencies to facilitate the effective linkages of service consumers with needed resources in other agencies.

Authority structures provide the sanction to ensure that environmentally oriented goals will be achieved by allocating power and authority to specific staff to enable them to carry out the tasks involved in meeting environmental objectives. An example is the allocation of authority to a staff member to negotiate affiliation agreements with other agencies. Given the probability that environmentally oriented goals will need to be given priority over people-change objectives, it is important to design the authority structures in such a way as to provide the sanction and support needed to achieve these goals. In the case, the supervisor had the authority to influence the worker to change to an environmental mode of intervention in serving the Smith family.

Reward structures specify the criteria for distribution of rewards and sanctions in an agency, such as promotions and disciplinary actions. Successful development of environmentally oriented programs is facilitated if reward systems reinforce staff behaviors that support this goal, while using sanctions to minimize lack of compliance. Such a system is illustrated in the case where the supervisor used performance evaluations to influence the worker to engage in environmental practice.

Interorganizational Relations structures specify the type of interactions that are expected with other agencies. Patterns of interorganizational relations vary from open and extensive relations and interdependence to a constrained and limited interrelations. Environmental practice necessitates extensive relations among agencies in order to assure that service users can obtain resources that might not be available in a single organization. Prior design of these relations is accomplished through the establishment of formal affiliation agreements between agencies that require each other's resources. In the case situation, the administrator took responsibility for developing an affiliation agreement with the school system in order to remove the obstacles to implementing the child abuse law.

Program Implementation. Program implementation by direct-service agency administrators consists first of the recruitment and selection of staff with personal and professional environmentally oriented goals and skills. This is reinforced and enhanced by in-service training and supervisory support and direction. Monitoring of program performance to determine whether the actual programs fulfill the environmental practice criteria is essential. For example, PASS and MEAP can be used to determine whether the program meets normalization and positive physical and social environmental standards.

In the case situation, the administrator directed recruitment and selection policies toward the hiring of environmentally trained staff. The supervisor's monitoring and supervision of staff in accordance with environmental standards was essential to insure that the agency goals were being implemented.

Community Arena

The community arena of environmental practice is concerned with community organization in social advocacy agencies and needs assessment and resource allocation in community planning agencies.

Micro Level: Social Advocacy

Advocacy for individual service users has previously been discussed under micro practice in direct-service organizations. Micro environmental practice in the community arena involves social advocacy on behalf of groups of service consumers. A similar distinction is made between case and cause advocacy (Kirst-Ashman and Hull 1993:466-468). Community organizers work in advocacy agencies by aiding in the organization of *groups* of service users/citizens to influence policymakers to remedy the gaps between community need and resources. Although Rothman (1979) separates locality development and organization from social action, these two arenas are combined here on the basis that they both involve representation of the interests of groups of citizens and service users. This type of micro practice typically occurs in community development and consumer advocacy agencies. Community development emphasizes social change through self-help, while social action uses conflict strategies to accomplish environmental change (Perlman and Gurin 1972:101). In the case, the role of the social action agency in advocating for more adequate housing for low-income citizens influenced the community planning agency to meet with the planning board. (See Chapter 4 for a discussion of the professional risks associated with advocacy.)

Macro Level: Community Planning

Macro practice on the community level involves community planning, with a focus on three functions: community needs assessment; facilitation of interagency coordination, and monitoring and feedback. A primary objective of community planners is to determine if community needs are being met by existing resources and, if not, to facilitate the development of these resources.

Community Needs Assessment. Community planners assess community needs to determine whether there is a gap between need and resources. It is important that the determination of community need not be overly influenced by existing service-delivery patterns. It is incorrect to assume that "more is better" if existing service-delivery modalities cannot meet community need (Rein 1969).

Five approaches to assessing community need have been identified: key informant; community forum; rates under treatment social indicators, and field survey (Warheit et al. 1978). The *key informant* approach to community need involves gathering information from persons who are knowledgeable about the community's needs and service utilization patterns. Persons normally selected as key informants are public officials and administrative and program personnel in human service agencies. Service consumers (current and former) are also a good source of information on service gaps. The *commu-*

nity forum approach involves the conducting of public meetings to which all residents are invited and where they express their beliefs about the needs and service patterns of the community. The *rates under treatment* method uses statistics of current service use to estimate community need and service patterns. The *social indicators* approach infers community need from such statistics as housing patterns, morbidity and mortality rates, age, sex, income, crime rates, housing conditions, and economic conditions. Finally, the *field survey* approach involves gathering data from a survey of a representative sample of the population regarding their health and well-being, as well as the pattern of service being received.

These different approaches to community needs assessment each have their own advantages and disadvantages. For example, the key informant approach has the advantage of opening lines of communication among human service agencies, but has the disadvantage of bias of informants based on individual or organizational priorities. The community forum method has the advantage of identifying interested citizens for future involvement, but the disadvantage rests with the difficulty of gaining a representative attendance at meetings. The rates under treatment approach has the advantage of having readily available and inexpensive data, but it also has the problem of achieving a representative sample. In contrast, the social indicators approach has the advantage of being able to compare the data with other communities, but the disadvantage that the indicators are only indirect measures of need. Finally, the field survey has the advantage of being scientifically valid and reliable, but the disadvantage of being more expensive than the other approaches.

In the case situation, the community planning agency obtained data on rates under treatment from the child welfare agency, which demonstrated the impact that lack of housing has on child abuse and the breakup of families. Community needs encompass interests of the total community, but particular emphasis is placed on the social problems of disadvantaged groups. This is crucial to achieving community integration needed to deal with such problems of chronic mental, physical, and social disability.

Community social planners must therefore have a broad view of community need based on the understanding that interests of various subgroups in the community are interdependent. An example is the contribution of community social planners to the integration of physical and social planning (Gans 1963; Perlman and Gurin 1972:240). Environmental protection statutes require environmental impact studies before approval is given to major programs of urban removal and highway construction. Social planners can contribute to environmental impact analyses by contributing their knowledge of the *social impact* of these planned changes in the physical environment. Lack of integration of physical and social planning is evident in urban renewal projects of the 1950's (Perlman and Gurin 1972:246; Wilson 1966). Perlman and Gurin (1972:242-244, 250-255) points to the planning of new towns and the Model Cities program are examples of a comprehensive approach to the integration of physical and social planning.

The role that a community social planner can play in facilitating the integration of social and physical planning is evident in the Smith case, the community planner was able to influence the urban renewal plans to include provision for low-income housing.

Facilitation of Inter-Agency Coordination. Community planning and allocating organizations have traditionally had a mandate to coordinate the agencies that they fund. However, these planning agencies are constrained by their "federated" structure (i.e., allocating boards represent provider agencies) from influencing provider agencies to engage in change (Rein and Morris 1962).

Given this constraint, social planners operating under the auspices of community planning and allocating agencies can facilitate interagency cooperation and coordination. Utilizing interorganizational exchange theory and community power structure concepts, they can facilitate formal compacts between organizations to accomplish program coordination and integration. More specifically, community planners can facilitate interagency coordination by acting as consultants to provider agencies and making them aware of their *interdependencies* based on shared goals and opportunities for resource exchange (Reid 1965). The role of the community planner in facilitating coordination between agencies was evident in the case, where the planner arranged for meetings of the directors of the housing authority and the public child welfare agency to plan for an affiliation agreement between the two agencies.

Monitoring and Feedback. Monitoring of the activities of pro-vider agencies to determine if they are meeting program objectives is intrinsic to the planning and allocation functions of community planning organizations (Perlman and Gurin 1972:226-233). The accountability function of community planning agencies requires them to obtain data on the programs that they fund. When programs are not meeting required objectives, it is the responsibility of the community planner to route this information to provider agencies so that they can modify their programs. This was illustrated in the case when the community planner provided information to the housing authority to show them that their policies were detrimental to single-parent families.

Societal Arena: Social Policy Formulating Agencies

Micro Level: Legislative Aide

The goal of micro practice in social policy formulating agencies is the linkage between service users/citizens and their legislative representatives. Typically, a legislative aide will have access to citizens through "hot lines" in the offices of legislators or the central offices of state and federal agencies. Historically, this func-tion was performed by the "ward heeler," who gave local citizens direct access to their political representatives. Citizen complaints and problems are dealt with in a manner similar to that of a case manager, with the potential for feedback to the representative to influence legislative and administrative policies related to the par-ticular social problem. For example, a director's hot line in a state public child welfare program provided service users and citizens with a means of both receiving individual aid and influencing ad-ministrative policies. An illustration of the latter was the change in the reimbursement policy for foster parents (McGuire 1995). In the Smith case, the complaints received in the office of the state legisla-tor about the failure of agencies to help citizens obtain needed resources were handled by a legislative aide. Feedback of this in-formation to the state legislator helped reinforce the need for a change in the state law.

Macro Level: Social Policy Analyst

Environmental practice in policy formulating agencies is directed at policies concerned with needs of such service consumer groups as the severely emotionally and physically disabled. Practice in this arena influences legislative and administrative policies on local, state, and federal levels. Practitioners function as aides to legislators and in staff roles in federal and state agencies that have responsibility for formulating social welfare policies. Substantive knowledge is required in the areas of social welfare policy that address the multiple needs of the severely disabled, such as housing, employment, income maintenance, and other survival services. The policy analyst requires analytical tools to accomplish policy formulation. The following policy analysis framework can facilitate such analytical work.

POLICY ANALYSIS FRAMEWORK

The framework for policy analysis used here draws on the Katz and Kahn model (1978:479-480,515-516), which assumes that the goal of policy formulation is major system change. Two kinds of change are possible: (1) changes in substantive goals, and (2) changes in strategies for achieving these goals.

Changes in Substantive Goals

The goals of a social program should be differentiated from its ultimate mission of service user benefit. Service consumer benefit in the area of environmental practice is operationalized by a positive change in the status of those who lack the resources to deal with the demands of life. Thus, the overall mission of human service programs is the improvement of the quality of life of persons who are in distress and suffer from such social problems as mental illness, poverty, mental retardation, ill health, problems of old age, crime, child abuse and neglect, inadequate housing, etc.

The goals of social programs have been classified into three categories: social care, social control, and rehabilitation (Neugeboren 1991:1-21). These goals are the means for achieving the mission of service user benefit. Clarity of this means-ends relationship is needed in order to ensure that service consumer benefit remains the primary purpose of human service programs.

The distinction among these three goals of human service programs (care, control, and rehabilitation) rests on the focus of intervention. *Social care* is concerned with changing the situations or environments of service consumers. It is the prime goal of environmental practice. *Rehabilitation,* in contrast, is directed at changing the individual service user. This goal is the predominant objective of human service programs. *Social control* is concerned with containment of individual deviancy. It is the "hidden agenda" of human service programs.

The policy analyst needs to understand the differences between these three goals because often they are interrelated (Neugeboren 1991:8-11). For example, rehabilitation of a service consumer can have the objective of the individual changing his/her environment. Policy formulation requires an understanding of the goals of human service programs, since it is directed at bringing about change in these substantive goals. This change can occur in four ways: (1) goal clarification, (2) shift in goal priorities, (3) addition of new goals, and (4) shift in mission.

Goal clarification is the process of assessing the relationship between the means and ends of human service programs. The purpose of goal clarification is to avoid goal displacement, whereby the means become ends unto themselves. For example, in the case situation, the child abuse statute advocated "treatment" (rehabilitation) as the means for reducing child abuse. The process of goal clarification would assess the relevance of this type of means for accomplishing the goal of reduced child abuse. Clarification could result in an analysis of the relevance of environmental factors (e.g., lack of adequate housing) as a significant influence contributing to child abuse. Recognition of environmental causes of child abuse would lead to a change in the statute emphasizing situational interventions as the preferred means for achieving the end of reduction of child abuse.

A *shift in goal priorities* involves a change in the rank order preference of the goals of a policy. The *addition of new goals* simply means that goals not previously included would be added. A *shift of mission* requires a dramatic change in direction of a program. This would be illustrated in child welfare policy if the treatment goal was replaced by the goal of environmental change.

Changes in Strategies for Achieving Goals

Changes in strategies for achieving goals can involve (1) alterations in the internal structural arrangements, and/or (2) changes in the manner in which an organization approaches its relationship with its external environment.

Internal Change

Internal change can be directed at structural change and/or methods for organizational assessment. An example of structural change is the movement between centralization vs. decentralization of service-delivery systems. Historically, there have been shifts from one strategy to the other, since there are costs and benefits associated with both strategies. Centralization results in greater control, but also in less responsiveness to local needs and greater insulation from local political forces (Hudson 1990:113). Decentralization moves power and control to those closest to the problem, but also creates greater vulnerablility to local political pressures.

In recent years, policy formulation has remained centralized, in contrast to policy implementation, which has become decentralized (Perrow 1976). Policymakers have recognized the need to decentralize agency structures to achieve more effective delivery of services. Critics argue that decentralization can result in such service-delivery problems, as specialization and selectivity loss of effective advocacy (Sosin 1990). The emphasis of environmental programs on the local community's responsibility to integrate the seriously disabled illustrates the need for decentralization of service delivery. Policy formulation in this regard would require that legislation and regulations dealing with the implemention of programs for the disabled, provide a mandate supporting local community control of service delivery for the disabled.

Another policy issue that is a potential area of strategy change is the alternative approaches of institutional vs. community care of the disabled. Cost/benefit comparisons suggest that community care can be more effective and efficient (Kam-Fong Monit Cheung 1988; Motwani and Herring 1988; Stein, Test, and Marx 1975). This has implications for policy formulation of programs for the severely disabled.

Organizational Assessment. Two contrasting strategies are possible in regard to policies concerned with program evaluation: (1) objective assessment or (2) self-fulfilling prophecy. Objective assessment involves the use of systematic procedures to determine whether or not a policy is achieving its goals of service consumer benefit. A self-fulfilling prophecy is strategy that assumes a policy is effective if its programs are in demand. Objective assessment in the child protection area would be determined by the reduction in child abuse or measurements of child functioning. In the case situation, the policy analyst determined that objective data was not routinely collected to evaluate the effectiveness of the child abuse statute. A policy change would develop a system for objective assessment to determine whether the law was achieving its purpose.

External Change

Strategies for change in external relations fall into two general categories: closed- and open-system strategies. Closed-system strategies assume that human service agencies can function independently of other organizations. In contrast, an open-system strategy views agencies as being interdependent. In the field of environmental practice, it is assumed that the complexity of service user needs obligate agencies to work together to pool their resources in order to achieve service consumer benefit. The policy analyst in the case situation could have proposed a change in the regulations to implement the child abuse law to include provision for interagency cooperation and coordination.

INTEGRATION OF MICRO AND MACRO ENVIRONMENTAL PRACTICE

As previously suggested, there are important interrelationships between the micro and macro levels of environmental practice.

Generalist practice models have attempted, with limited success, to integrate both micro and macro practice. Rothman suggests that practitioners serving highly vulnerable populations need expertise on "both sides of the psychosocial fence," requiring a broader social context in formulating individual service plans (Rothman 1994:14). In our discussion of the relationship between micro and macro environmental practice we have emphasized that although there are similarities between these two levels of practice, an important distinction is that the micro level focuses on changing individuals while the macro seeks to change systems. These different functions of micro and macro practitioners result in disparities of authority and power between the two levels. An awareness of this power structure is required in order to understand the relationships between the levels and the potential for integration of micro and macro environmental practice.

Common and Specific Knowledge and Skill

Underlying the connections between micro and macro environmental practice is the knowledge and skills that are *common or specific* to the two levels. As indicated previously, some would claim that dividing practice into micro and macro areas is creating a false dichotomy, while others assert that there are significant differences. Knowing the similarities and differences of micro and macro practice will enable us to clarify the links between these types of practice.

Practitioners at both levels share a common conceptual knowledge base which rests on the use of social structural concepts such as intraorganizational bureaucratic and systems theories, interorganizational exchange concepts, community power structure, and social change theories. In the case situation, the micro worker would use understanding of bureaucratic structure to impact on the school system's low expectation of Mary Jane. On the macro level, the administrator used social exchange concepts to develop an affiliation agreement with the school system.

As previously suggested the practice skills common to micro and macro environmental practice are sociopolitical in nature. The common skills include decision making, negotiating, representing, staffing, leadership, and monitoring.

The specific knowledge and skills of micro and macro environmental practice relate to the different targets of practice intervention: the individual service users' situation in micro practice and agency structures and policies in macro practice. Although both interventions are concerned with service consumer benefit, the goal of changing service consumers' situations requires different strategies (e.g., how to make better *use* of existing policies to achieve individual service user benefit) than those related to the macro goal of changing policies that affect all service consumers (e.g., influencing the power structure to change policy).

Cooperation vs. Conflict Between Micro and Macro Practitioners

It is debated whether micro and macro environmental practitioners can *cooperate* or whether there are *inevitable strains*. Frequent tensions between direct service workers and administrators has been attributed to differences in orientations stemming from the micro professional's requirement for autonomy and the macro practitioner's need to exert authority and control (Patti and Austin 1977). However, cooperation between these two levels is possible if there is an understanding that both share the goal of service consumer benefit (Neugeboren 1991:136). The micro professional could be given the autonomy to have control over the *means* for achieving service user benefit while granting the administrator the authority to have control over the *outcomes* of service consumer benefit.

Interdependency Between Micro and Macro Practice

Linkage between micro and macro practice is facilitated by the interdependency between the two levels. In addition to the shared goal of service consumers benefit, this interdependency stems from shared needs for information and support. Two-way communication of information between micro and macro practitioners is required to facilitate both kinds of practice. Administrators, planners, and policymakers need information from direct service practitioners about the barriers to effective service. This feedback can be used to evaluate policy in terms of equity, efficiency, and effectiveness, as was illustrated in the case where the direct-service workers communicated with the administrator the problems involved in working with the school system.

Communication from macro to micro practitioners is required to help the direct practitioner to appreciate the rationale for how policies are to achieve collective consumer benefit, also formulated in terms of equity, efficiency, and effectiveness.

Interdependency between micro and macro practice stems in part from direct practitioners' need for sanction and support for their intervention actions. This is particularly true for interagency case coordination, which requires interagency affiliation agreements, as illustrated in the case situation with regard to work with the school system.

The integration of micro and macro practice will be a theme running throughout this book. This linkage will be discussed in various environmental practice areas, such as community resource coordination, social support, organizational environments, and practice with severely disabled.

PRACTICE SKILLS

Environmental practice on micro and macro levels in the organizational, community, and societal arenas requires particular practice skills. These skills are: (1) decision making; (2) monitoring; (3) leadership; (4) negotiating; (5) staffing; and (6) representing. In this chapter, these skills will be briefly defined and applied to environmental practice situations on the micro and macro levels and in the three arenas of practice. Practice skills will be discussed in more detail in Chapter 3, as well as applied and illustrated in environmental practice situations throughout the book.

Although skills are partly a matter of individual practitioner competencies, it should be kept in mind that the organizational context influences how, when, and where these skills can be effectively applied (Weiss 1972:113-121). Kennedy (1980) suggests that success in industry requires not only technical expertise, but also *political* skills (Gummer 1990; Jansson 1984). The following chart provides the definitions of practice skills needed for environmental practice.

PRACTICE SKILLS	DEFINITION
Decision Making	Problem solving–analyze cause and determine solutions
Monitoring	Verify achievement of objectives
Leadership	Influence behavior
Negotiating	Coordinate interdependent units
Staffing	Integrate individual and system goals
Representing	Sell agency programs

Practice Skills in Direct Practice, Administration, Planning, and Policy

The above skills are relevant for environmental practice on the micro and macro levels, as well as in the various arenas of practice. *Decision-making* skills are used by direct-service practitioners in analyzing case situations to formulate service objectives. On the macro level, administrators use this skill to analyze agency problems and to formulae appropriate solutions. Community planners use decision-making skills in analyzing community need and determining the most appropriate means for meeting this need. Policy analysts use a decision-making procedure involving problem formulation, the evaluation of alternative solutions to arrive at an optimum policy solution (Kahn 1969).

In the Smith case, the caseworker used decision-making skills in developing a case plan for Mary Jane. The supervisor also used a decision-making procedure to develop a plan for the family, but arrived at a different determination than the caseworker, concluding that lack of housing was a key factor contributing to the abuse problem. The policy analyst in the state central office also used decision-making skills that led to the revision of the regulations for the hiring of child protection staff.

Monitoring skills also are applicable to both micro and macro environmental practice. Direct-service practitioners use this skill to achieve self-regulated practice by obtaining information on the results of their efforts to aid individual service users (Garvin and Seabury 1984:217-235; Taylor 1987). Administrators use monitoring skills to evaluate whether agency programs are achieving desired objectives (Patti 1983:36). Program monitoring is one of the prime functions associated with community planning (Perlman and

Gurin 1972:226-233). Policy analysts use monitoring skills to assess the effectiveness of existing policies in order to determine if changes are necessary (Jansson 1984:235-276).

In the case situation, the administrator monitored the agency practice of hiring clinically trained staff, which led to a change in this policy. The community planner used monitoring skills in obtaining statistics on the link between lack of housing and the incidence of child abuse. Similarly, the state policy analyst monitored the staffing of the child protection agency, leading to the revision of the hiring regulations.

Leadership is required on all levels and in all arenas of environmental practice. Leadership involves influencing others to perform above a minimum level (Katz and Kahn 1978: 528). Direct-service workers use this skill to gain the cooperation of superiors and colleagues, both in and outside of their agency, in order to enhance their ability to obtain resources for their service consumers. Administrators use leadership skills to influence staff to perform above the minimum level. Community planners need leadership skills to influence agencies to coordinate their services. Policy analysts use leadership skills to persuade policymakers to introduce new policies or modify existing ones.

In the case situation, leadership skills were evident in the supervisor's use of performance evaluation to influence the worker to move toward an environmentally oriented service delivery approach. The planner used leadership skills to influence the planning board to modify the urban renewal program so as to include low-income housing.

Negotiating skills facilitate the coordination of sub-units, whether they are different departments within an agency or autonomous organizations (Popple 1984). This skill utilizes the principle of social exchange in achieving cooperation. The direct-service environmental practitioner negotiates with staff from other agencies to link the service consumer with needed resources. Administrators use negotiating skills to obtain affiliation agreements with other agencies. Planners negotiate with agencies that they fund to insure that programs will maximize service user benefit. Policy analysts negotiate with legislators to influence them to formulate new policies or change old ones.

In the case situation, negotiating skills were used by the administrator to develop an affiliation agreement with the school system. The planner negotiated an agreement between the housing authority and the public child welfare agency.

Staffing skills involve the integration of staff and organizational goals. The direct-service worker uses staffing skills to achieve a closer fit between his/her personal and professional goals and the organization's purposes. Some of the mechanisms used in staffing are in-service training and role clarification. Administrators use staffing skills in the recruitment, selection, training, and evaluation of staff performance (Pecora and Austin 1987). Planners use staffing skills when influencing the agencies that they fund to implement appropriate recruitment, selection, training, and staff performance evaluation policies. Policy analysts also use these skills in formulating policies that facilitate the appropriate use of staff to achieve environmentally oriented service programs.

In the case situation, the supervisor used staffing skills in the utilization of a staff performance evaluation to help the worker move toward an environmentally oriented service. The policy analyst used staffing skills in the formulation of new regulations in the hiring of child protection workers.

Representing skills are also used in micro and macro environmental practice (Schneider & Sharon 1982). Representing skills come into use in efforts to sell a program to groups and individuals external to the organization. Direct-service practitioners use representing skills with staff from agencies with which they are attempting to develop linkage for their service consumers. Administrators use representing skills to obtain social support for and legitimation of the agency's programs from funding authorities and the general public. Similarly, community planners and policy analysts need representing skills when attempting to obtain community support and sanction for their programs.

In the case situation, the director used representing skills to convince the chairman of the state legislative committee to revise the child abuse law. The community planner used representing skills to influence the community planning board to modify the urban renewal plan.

SUMMARY

This chapter presented a conceptual framework that integrated levels of practice (micro and macro) with three arenas of practice: organization, community, and societal, while contrasting the micro level goal of changing service user situations with the macro level goal of changing policies. The influence of these different practice contexts was highlighted to indicate how they constrain or facilitate practice. In addition, seven practice skills for environmental practice on both the micro and macro levels of intervention were briefly defined. Throughout the chapter, the case situation presented in Chapter 1 was used to illustrate the conceptsin concrete terms.

STUDY QUESTIONS

1. You are a direct-service worker in the agency serving the Smith case. Indicate the kinds of environmental services you would provide.

2. As a direct-service practitioner in the Smith case, how would you decide whether to focus your intervention on the individuals or on the environment?

3. You are the director of the child welfare agency described in the case situation. What would you do to move the agency toward an environmentally oriented practice?

4. You are a policy analyst working for the state government. What actions would you take to promote programs with an environmental focus?

5. You are a community planner. How would you facilitate cooperation between agencies to better serve severely disabled service consumers?

6. You are a community organizer working in a social advocacy agency. Indicate the kinds of efforts you would make to achieve better services for child abuse service consumers.

PART II:
ENVIRONMENTAL PRACTICE
IN ACTION

Chapter 3

SKILLS IN ENVIRONMENTAL PRACTICE

Skills in Environmental Practice

INTRODUCTION

Environmental practice on micro and macro levels in the organizational, community, and societal arenas requires specific practice skills. These skills are: (1) decision making; (2) monitoring; (3) leadership; (4) negotiating; (5) staffing; and (6) representing (Schneider 1978). Each of these will be defined, discussed and applied to environmental practice situations throughout the book.

Although skills are related to individual practitioner competencies, contextual factors can influence how, when, and where these skills can be effectively applied. Context is important both within an organization and between organizations. For example, within organizations, the goals and philosophies of staff can constrain the use of monitoring skills (Weiss 1972:113-121). Between agencies, the self-interests of constituencies can influence the outcomes of negotiations (Lauffer 1984:104). In industrial settings, individual technical competence is insufficient for success—"political" skills are also required (Kennedy 1980).

This presentation of practice skills therefore includes not only the technical aspects, but also the situational contingencies that affect skill use. These skills will also be related to practice arenas in the roles performed by direct-service staff and administrators, community planners, social advocates, and policy analysts.

The following case situation illustrates the practice skills, contrasting technical and political skills and demonstrating commonality of micro and macro skills. The six practice skills will be discussed in terms of: (1) practice arenas; (2) technical aspects; and (3) situational influences, followed by a discussion of the interrelationship between the skills.

CASE: COMMUNITY CARE FOR THE SEVERELY DISABLED MENTALLY ILL

New State Policy

The lack of adequate community care for the severely mentally ill was highlighted by the publicity given in the media to homelessness in the cities of Central County. Politicians, business owners, and other prominent citizens demanded that the State Department of Mental Health take action to solve the problem.

Partially in response to community pressure, the department proposed a new policy requiring community mental health centers funded with state money to establish new programs to serve the severely mentally ill in the community. This new state policy initiative was also based on a study of mental health service delivery programs, which found that the severely mentally ill were under-served.

The State Department had considerable difficulty implementing the new regulations requiring community mental health centers to give priority to the severely mentally ill. These centers were committed to serving less-disturbed service users. The directors and boards of the community mental health centers used their political influence to thwart and delay the implementation of these regulations. Another major barrier to the execution of this new policy was the lack of trained professionals skilled in work with the severely mentally ill.

The mental health department instituted a public information program to educate the citizenry on the problem. A series of public meetings were held throughout the state to inform the public of the new policy, and a statewide citizen group was organized to advocate for community care of the mentally ill.

A policy analyst working in the State Department of Mental Health took action to remedy the lack of adequately trained staff. She approached the dean of the State School of Social Work with a proposal to fund a special program for educating BSW and MSW students in the skills needed to serve the severely mentally disabled. Although the dean supported this new educational effort, some of the clinically oriented faculty were unalterably opposed. Pressure generated by the State Department of Mental Health and the State Department of Higher Education resulted in the enactment of the training program.

County Planning

The county planning agency also participated in this new educational program. Through their funding of community service agencies, they influenced them to serve as training sites for student interns.

An agency needs-assessment study also determined that the mentally ill were underserved in Central County. It discovered that a lack of coordination between the county mental hospital and the county community mental health center (CCMHC) was one of the causes of the problem. Dr. Wilson, the community planner, arranged for a countywide meeting of human service providers to address the need for better coordination of service programs. The press was invited to this meeting and reported it in the newspaper the following day. Dr. Wilson also arranged for a televised panel interview on the subject of coordination of human service programs and invited a local councilman to participate.

After this publicity on the need for better agency coordination, Dr. Wilson met with the directors of the mental health center and the mental hospital to explain the planning agency's goal of interorganizational coordination. The media publicity stimulated interest in the possibilities for better coordination between their agencies. Subsequent meetings with Dr. Wilson led to an agreement between the mental health center and the mental hospital to establish joint case conferences on patients discharged into the community.

The CCMHC Takes Action

The CCMHC is responsible for providing comprehensive mental health services to all residents of the county. Public criticism was leveled at this agency for not adequately serving the mentally ill discharged from the county mental hospital. The CCMHC is a typical mental health center, serving primarily less-disabled emotionally disturbed patients with the use of psychotherapeutically oriented treatments. A new director, Dr. Margaret Smith, was hired under pressure from the state to make the necessary changes to increase service to the more severely disabled patients in the community.

The new director of CCMHC first determined the basis of the problem of lack of service to the severely mentally ill. She identified the following difficulties:

1. Lack of coordination of services with the county mental hospital.
2. CCMHC staff who were not interested nor trained in serving the severely mentally ill.

3. Poor coordination between the Partial Care and Counseling departments within the CCMHC.
4. Ineffective supervision at the CCMHC.
5. Poor public image of CCMHC.

Dr. Smith decided that she first had to concern herself with the lack of skilled staff. She recruited new direct-service staff who were given the responsibility of expediting referrals from the county mental hospital.

Dr. Smith then took steps to respond to the criticism that the CCMHC was not serving the needs of the severely mentally ill. She created a public relations department within CCMHC that distributed press releases and initiated a public speaking program before community groups. Information was presented on the problems associated with community care of the mentally disabled, including the lack of housing and employment. She also publicized the effort to coordinate services between the CCMHC and the county mental hospital.

The director also appointed new members of the board, including an influential businessman and a consumer representative. An educational program was instituted to acquaint the board members with the problems and issues surrounding the care of the mentally ill in the community. A technical advisory committee was created that included influential persons with the expertise to help solve some of the barriers to community care of mentally ill. A member from the real estate board assisted with the problems associated with the creation of group homes. A representative from the industrial labor council helped with the development of employment opportunities for the mentally disabled.

Program Assessment at the CCMHC

Dr. Smith, under pressure from the state, instituted a program-evaluation system to determine why the CCMHC was not serving the severely mentally ill. However, the staff resisted reporting information, since previous evaluation systems had been of little value to them in their practice. They were also concerned that the information could be used to evaluate individual work performance. Dr. Smith indicated in a staff meeting that only aggregated data would be collected, and therefore it could not be used for evaluation of individual staff performance. Staff were also informed that they would participate in the design of the evaluation system, including the development of criteria for case outcome. Subsequently, staff consensus was obtained on patient functioning in the community as the service outcome. The program evaluation would consist of a comparison of community adjustment of patients receiving different kinds of service interventions.

The information collected from the program monitoring system included the types of patients served and of services provided, as well as patient outcomes. The data corroborated earlier assessments of the overall lack of service to the severely disabled mentally ill at the CCMHC. An analysis of the factors associated with effective service to the severely disabled revealed that community resource coordination was more successful than therapeutic technologies in helping patients adjust in the community. It was also determined that community resource coordination consumed less staff time than therapy. This information was fed back to line staff, who subsequently supported the establishment of in-service training in community resource coordination.

CCMHC Staff Recruitment, Selection, and Evaluation

As indicated above, Dr. Smith gave priority to the hiring of new staff skilled in service to the severely mentally ill. She had her personnel director recruit social workers trained in community organization to fill the direct-service positions. The selection process used simulation tests that required the applicant to make case decisions in service to the severely mentally ill. Those applicants who favored such interventions as the provision of concrete resources (housing and employment) training were rated high in the selection process.

Clinically oriented staff had difficulty in accepting the new staff. They took the position that community resource coordination was a task that could be done by nonprofessionals, in contrast to counseling, which they felt required professional training. Dr. Smith dealt with this situation by establishing a separate community resource coordination unit that was given authority and status.

Dr. Smith also discovered that the middle managers were hiring direct-service staff who were clinically oriented and not interested in serving the severely mentally ill. She solved this problem by placing hiring responsibility with the personnel manager, who was directly supervised by Dr. Smith.

A staff performance-evaluation system was also instituted. It was found that the direct-service staff who were clinically trained were unskilled in the use of such interventions as self-help groups. The in-service training program was expanded to include different environmental interventions, such as referrals to self-help, housing, and employment resources. A merit system was also developed in conjunction with the performance-evaluation system. Although these staffing initiatives increased turnover of some clinical and administrative staff, they also resulted in more and better service to the severely disabled.

The staff-evaluation system revealed that line administrators favored supportive supervisory techniques and lacked the ability to direct their staff. Training in directive supervision was instituted, which was useful in educating the direct-service staff in environmental intervention skills.

Coordination Within the CCMHC

Dr. Smith discovered that the partial care department was not receiving referrals from the counseling department. Lack of agreement between the department heads on the kinds of services needed by the severely mentally ill was the underlying cause of the problem. The counseling chief believed that these patients needed therapy. The chief of the partial care department thought that vocational training was a more appropriate intervention. Dr. Smith took a firm position to convince these department heads that referrals to partial care could be made in conjunction with therapy. She persuaded them that vocational training and counseling interventions were compatible. She also pointed out that working together would provide opportunities for the two departments to share scarce office space.

Case Coordination Between the CCMHC and the County Mental Hospital

Ms. Jones, one of the newly recruited direct-service staff members at the CCMHC, soon discovered that no referrals were being received from the state hospital. She learned that some of the professional staff at the hospital were reluctant to discharge the severely disabled because they considered them "too sick" to live in the community.

Ms. Jones considered several solutions to this problem, including developing a relationship with one of the hospital social workers in order to facilitate case referrals and asking her supervisor to suggest that Dr. Smith address the problem with the hospital director. Ms. Jones decided to work with a hospital social worker, because this solution was one which she could implement herself immediately. However, Ms. Jones was careful to select a social worker at the hospital who accepted the value of community care for discharged patients.

Ms. Jones arranged a meeting with Ms. Williams, a direct-service worker at the county mental hospital, to discuss methods for increasing referrals from the hospital to the CCMHC. Prior to this meeting, the women agreed that they both shared the goal of helping the severely mentally ill patients adjust in the community. They also agreed that it would be useful for both parties to exchange information that might facilitate patient discharge and adjustment in the community.

Ms. Jones met with her supervisor prior to the meeting to do some planning. They agreed that the basic problem was how to expedite referrals from the hospital. They thought that although the hospital staff would be reluctant to have them become directly involved in their operations, they might agree to share information, since they were under pressure from the Central Office of the Department of Mental Health to coordinate their services with the CCMHC. However, the CCMHC was also aware that they were at a disadvantage in their ability to influence the hospital, since they had no direct authority over the hospital.

An essential goal of the negotiations was to obtain information early in the discharge process so that the CCMHC would have the time to plan for appropriate community interventions. The negotiating plan called for Ms. Jones to initiate discussions by requesting participation in the discharge planning meetings at the hospital, with the knowledge that this demand, although desirable, could be traded for a lesser demand of receiving two weeks notice of impending discharges. Either outcome would provide sufficient time and information to allow the CCMHC to plan for community placement. It was also decided that the meeting should take place at the hospital. This meeting site would allow Ms. Jones to use an adjournment strategy to provide her time to consult with her supervisor.

At the meeting, Ms. Jones first requested her participation in discharge planning meetings at the hospital. This demand was unacceptable to Ms. Williams, who lacked the authority to agree to this request. Ms. Williams countered by requesting a role in the aftercare of patients being discharged. This demand was rejected by Ms. Jones. The meeting was adjourned so that both parties could consult with their respective supervisors. They agreed to meet again in a week.

Ms. Jones was informed by her supervisor that it would not be possible for the hospital social worker to participate in the aftercare program at the CCMHC. The two agreed that if it was not possible to gain participation in hospital case conferences, then Ms. Jones should demand two week's prior notification by the hospital of patients being discharged.

At the second meeting, Ms. Jones continued to make the demand for participation in hospital case conferences. Ms. Williams pressed for a hospital role in the CCMHC aftercare program. An impasse was reached. Ms. Williams fell back to a position of a hospital role in CCMHC case conferences. This was rejected by Ms. Jones, who countered with a demand for a four-week notification procedure. They finally agreed on a two-week notification process. A follow-up meeting formulated the details for implementing the plan for the two-week notice of discharge, including the provision of specific information on patients to the CCMHC.

ISSUES

Two issues central to the use of skills in environmental practice are: (1) the influence of situational and political factors, and (2) the commonality of micro and macro skills in this area of human service practice.

Technical vs. Political Skills

Skills are assumed to be dependent on individual abilities. Competence in such varied areas as sports, the arts, or the helping professions requires the mastery of specific sets of individual behaviors in order to produce definable results. This minimizes the influence of external forces on successful skill performance. However, even in sports, situational factors can affect performance, as in the case of the person who performs well in practice but does not do as well under the pressure of competition (Ryan 1958:123).

The stress on individualism in American culture downplays the effects of environmental factors on human functioning. The belief that the individual is responsible for his/her destiny is evident in the focus of human service practice on personality as the key to successful functioning. This is also evident in the political arena, where "strength of character" is emphasized. Media campaigns in U.S. presidential elections promote those individual traits that the public believes are associated with competence. However, when situations change, such as the death of an incumbent, and the individual is forced into a leadership role, a person who seems rather ordinary may rise to the occasion and exhibit skills and abilities not previously appreciated. An example of this is seen in the case of President Harry Truman.

In the human service professions, with their stress on the individual as the cause and solution of social problems (Neugeboren 1991:239), there is particular need to appreciate environmental influences on practitioner performance. For example, the success of program monitoring depends on more than technical data collection skills. Successful data collection also depends on an understanding of staff reactions to the monitoring efforts and the use of strategies to overcome staff resistance. Therefore, throughout this chapter on practice skills, consideration will be given to how situational factors can effect the skill performance of practitioners.

Commonality of Micro and Macro Skills

As indicated in Chapter 1, environmental practice occurs on both a micro and a macro level in the three practice arenas. The six practice skills used in these practice arenas are relevant for both micro and macro practitioners. Skills such as decision making, monitoring, staffing, negotiating, leadership, and representing are usually associated with macro practice, since environmental manipulations require skills that are somewhat different than those needed for changing people. As indicated previously, influencing environments requires use of sociopolitical skills in contrast with socio-emotional interventions in people-changing practice. But the six practice skills are also applicable to direct service practice. Therefore, throughout the book, these six skills will be applied to both macro and micro practice situations.

In Chapter 1, the integration of micro and macro practice was presented as a theme of this book. The proposition that there are skills common to both micro and macro environmental practice further advances the potential for an integrated practice even though the actual application of these skills will vary with situational contexts.

DEFINITIONS OF PRACTICE SKILLS

The six practice skills will be discussed first in terms of how they are used in the three practice arenas. The specification of the technical aspects of these skills will follow, concluding with the presentation of the situational influences on the use of these skills. The case presented earlier in the chapter will be used to illustrate the applicability of these skills in practice.

Decision Making

Decision making is a procedure that uses rationality in formulating problems, searching for alternative solutions, and arriving at a decision after considering the relative costs and benefits of different alternatives. However, such nonrational contextual factors as the organizations' goals, structures, auspices, and technologies can constrain or facilitate rationality in the decision-making process (Neugeboren 1991:169-174; Perlman and Gurin 1972:75-83). Therefore, decision making is conceived as involving both rational stages and nonrational situational factors that hinder or promote an effective problem-solving process (Katz and Kahn 1978:487-501).

Decision Making in Arenas of Environmental Practice

Decision-making skill is intrinsic to both macro and micro environmental practice interventions. In direct practice, case decision making requires a systematic approach to analyzing service consumer needs, searching for the most appropriate environmental solution, and obtaining feedback from the service user on the results of the decision. In the above case, Ms. Jones, the direct-service worker at CCMHC, engaged in a decision-making procedure in analyzing and solving the problem of case referrals from the county mental hospital.

At the macro level, administrators of direct-service agencies use decision making in management tasks. For example, budgeting is a decision making tool that helps transform goals into service realities (Lewis and Lewis 1983:51-73). The design of organizational structures by administrators is also dependent on decision-making skills. Specifying role, communication, reward, authority, and interorganizational arrangements and different subsystem structures and functions (Neugeboren 1991:55-88) requires decisions as to which structures are functional for agency goals. The case illustrates the director's need to make a variety of decisions, including hiring of new staff and instituting program-evaluation, performance-appraisal, and training systems.

Decision making is also relevant for the community planner (Ehlers, Austin, and Prothero 1976:81-114; Lewis and Lewis 1983: 20-50; Perlman and Gurin 1972:61-75) when assessing community. Social advocates use decision-making skills in determining the best strategies for representing service consumer groups.

In the societal arena, policy analysts use decision making in the policy formulation process. This includes defining needs, analyzing policy alternatives, and deciding which policy will meet the defined need (Kahn 1969). Decision making also comes into play in the enactment of regulations to implement policies.

In the case situation, the planner used a decision-making process to facilitate better coordination of services between the CCMHC and the county mental hospital. The policy analyst in the Department of Mental Health used decision-making skills in the enactment of regulations to implement the new state policy requiring mental health centers to give priority service to the severely mentally ill.

Technical Aspects

The technical aspects of decision making will be discussed in terms of the rational stages of the problem-solving process. The nonrational organizational factors in the decision making process will be included in the section on situational influences on this skill area.

Rational Stages. Rational decision making involves five sequential stages: (1) determination of immediate pressures; (2) problem formulation; (3) search for alternative solutions; (4) cost/benefit evaluation of alternatives and selection of the most desirable solution; and (5) obtaining feedback on the consequences of the decision.

Decisions in human service practice are made out of necessity. Practitioners are required to act because of various *pressures* on them to solve problems. These pressures may stem from the professional's own conviction that a change is needed to enhance service user benefit. Often the dominant pressure for decisions is external to the individual decision maker, coming from service consumers, staff within ones agency, or persons in other organizations. These pressures can influence the decision maker to skip some steps in the process and move to premature action without considering alternative solutions and their consequences.

The second stage of the rational process of decision making involves *problem formulation.* A comprehensive approach to problem definition requires that information be obtained from multiple sources, to insure that one is aware of different perspectives on problem causes and solutions. Problem definitions are intrinsically linked to ideological beliefs on causality of human problems (Neugeboren 1991:227-248). Decision making in environmental practice requires particular attention to *situational* causes of problems.

The *search for solutions,* the third stage of the decision making procedure, requires that a broad range of alternatives be considered. As suggested above, this can be achieved by the decision maker seeking out perspectives from different persons in and outside the agency. In general, solutions that have been used in the past will be given preference over novel ones. Problem solvers will seek solutions within existing policies, rather than resorting to the formulation of new policies.

Evaluation of anticipated consequences of alternative solutions involves comparing the costs and benefits of different alternatives before arriving at a decision. Central to this assessment is the outcome goal of service consumer benefit. The costs and benefits of different alternatives have to be determined in terms of the consequences for service user interests.

The final stage of the rational decision-making process is *feedback from service consumers on the consequences of the decision.* This requires a method of obtaining information on the results of the decision to determine if unanticipated consequences require further action (see selection on Monitoring below).

Situational Influences

The five stages of rational decision making are influenced by nonrational situational factors, including: (1) problem-solving dilemmas; (2) organizational context; and (3) bounded rationality. These factors can constrain and/or facilitate a rational problem solving process. These nonrational factors constitute the "decision environment." The decision maker must make an effort to be logical and rational within the boundaries of this situational context.

Problems are solved by use of past precedent derived from existing policies. When a difficulty cannot be resolved by use of existing rules and procedures we are confronted with a *dilemma,* which requires a reformulation of existing policies to solve the problem. Human service policies often assume that the cause of service consumers's difficulties lie within the individual. Environmental practitioners who are aware of situational causes may therefore be confronted with dilemmas that require new approaches that rest outside of existing policies.

The *organizational context* also constrains/facilitates the process of rational decision making. This context includes the auspices, goals, structures, ideologies, and technologies of the system. Problem formulation, the search for solutions, and evaluation of alternatives will be influenced by the nature of this context. For example, an agency goal of changing service consumer attitudes and behavior will constrain a practitioner from pursing an environmental change intervention.

The last nonrational element that influences rational decision making is *bounded rationality.* This factor results in a simplified trial-and-error method of decision making where optimization is replaced by mere satisfaction. The more complex and time-consuming rational approach to problem solving, is replaced by a more expedient trial-and-error method. Similarly, *optimal* solutions, which may require change in status quo and disturb the equilibrium of the system, are replaced by *satisfactory* solutions ("satisficing") that are acceptable to persons in the system.

As indicated, different agency auspices can influence practice. This occurs in the area of planning, where diverse contexts have different task requirements. Voluntary organizations, service agencies, and planning organizations, because of the varying goals and structures of their particular sponsors, place different demands on the planner practitioner (Perlman and Gurin 1972:75-83). The public or private nature of agency sponsorship will have different effects on service delivery patterns (Neugeboren 1970a).

Both the operation of rational decision making and the influence of nonrational situational factors were evident in the case situation. Ms. Jones followed the stages of rational decision making in the solution of the problem of lack of referrals from the mental hospital. After defining the problem, she systematically searched for alternative solutions and did a comparative evaluation of the consequences of each solution. She decided that the best solution to the problem was to develop a working relationship with a hospital social worker.

In contrast, Dr. Smith circumvented this rational procedure in making the decision to recruit new direct-service staff. Under pressure from the Department of Mental Health to make quick changes in the agency, she selected an alternative solution that seemed the least difficult to enact. She "satisficed" by avoiding dealing with the problem of middle managers and line supervisors.

The constraining influence of the system context also is evident in the case situation. The policy analyst in Department of Mental Health was constrained in implementing the new policy of priority for service to the severely mentally ill by the ideological and political forces in the mental health system. The people-change clinical bias and the power of the community mental health centers also had to be considered in the decision making of the direct-service worker, administrator, and planner.

Monitoring

Monitoring involves *verifying* whether an agency is accomplishing established objectives. It is an information-based technology that requires skill in data collection, processing, and dissemination in a manner that facilitates micro and macro environmental practice. Although monitoring traditionally provides information for program accountability, it can provide important purpose of feedback to macro and micro practitioners to help steer their actions (Taylor 1987; Weissman 1977). Integrated information systems designed to meet the complementary needs of both direct-service and administration have been proposed (Mutschler and Hasenfeld 1986). Monitoring is directed at correcting system deficiencies, rather than at evaluating individual staff performance, which is a staffing function.

Monitoring in Arenas of Environmental Practice

Monitoring skills are an integral part of environmental practice. Direct-service practitioners use feedback on their efforts to modify their interventions and make them more efficient and effective (Briar and Blythe 1985; Nurius and Hudson 1988). Administrators monitor direct-service programs to determine if they are achieving their intended ends (Phillips, Dimsdale, and Taft 1985). Monitoring influences their decision making on resource allocations, staffing patterns, and the continuation, elimination, or expansion of programs (Rapp 1984:74-76).

Community planners monitor the programs they fund (Kettner and Martin 1985; Perlman and Gurin 1972:226-233). Using data on the accomplishments of these programs, they make decisions as to whether funding should be continued or reallocated to other, more-effective programs. Planners focus on how the accomplishments of particular agencies fit into the more comprehensive community planning goals of reducing service fragmentation and enhancing service continuity and integration. Community planners will monitor services delivered to different population groups to verify whether previously established standards are being met for these groups (Poertner and Rapp 1985). Social advocates use monitoring skills in compiling information from service user groups for feedback to administrators. Policy analysts use information obtained from systematic monitoring efforts to decide whether policies should be continued or changed.

The case situation illustrates the use of monitoring by the direct-service staff, the administrator, the planner, and the policy analyst. Feedback that showed that community resource coordination was an effective technology helped produce a modification of the service interventions of the direct-service workers. It also guided the administrator to enact in-service training in this service methodology and to recruit new staff trained in this area.

Data from a monitoring study conducted by the county planning agency on the lack of coordination between the county mental hospital and the CCMHC was instrumental in facilitating the role of community planner in promoting linkage between these two organizations. The statewide monitoring study, which discovered that the severely mentally ill were being underserved, was used as the basis for the new policy initiative.

Technical Aspects

Monitoring is directed at evaluation of effort, efficiency, and/or effectiveness (Tripody, Fellin, Epstein 1978). Monitoring of program *effort* verifies whether service interventions and structures are implemented in accordance with established standards. It focuses on the activities and tasks performed by staff. Environmental interventions, including practice skills discussed throughout this book, are examples of program efforts that may be monitored.

Evaluation of program *efficiency* focuses on the costs of service. Since service costs are mostly tied to utilization of staff time, time-measuring skills are used in this monitoring area. Time-sampling systems are devised to assemble information on the amount of time devoted to different staff activities.

Monitoring for program *effectiveness* involves technical procedures for service user impact evaluation (Lewis and Lewis 1983:144-172; Ehlers, Austin, and Prothero 1976:337-377; Patti, Poertner, and Rapp 1987; Rapp and Poertner 1992). This requires skill in the systematic design of systems for measuring program input in relation to outcomes of service consumer benefit. The purpose of effectiveness evaluations is to determine *if* and *why* programs are or are not successful. Thus, effectiveness monitoring is not only concerned with the results of programs, but also with the kinds of program structures that lead to outcomes of service user benefit (Patti, Poertner, and Rapp 1987:15-17; Rubin 1985). Successful effectiveness monitoring depends on the understanding that holding line professionals accountable for results without giving them the kind of information that will help them improve their performance can lead to sabotage of the monitoring program (Rapp and Anderson 1975).

Monitoring requires technical ability to create systematic and *useful* procedures for the design and implementation of evaluation projects. There is evidence that managers and practitioners do not find performance information reports useful in guiding them in day-to-day practice (Nurius and Hudson 1988:359; Neugeboren 1993; Poertner and Rapp 1980: Rapp 1984:71). Computerized information systems have the potential for producing *too much* data, leading to information overload (Mutschler and Cnaan 1985; Rapp 1984:70). Therefore, monitoring requires skill in producing usable reports that employ a variety of communication tools, such as numbers, words, and visual charts (Neugeboren 1957; Nurius and Hudson 1988:395) that provide the practitioner with *timely* information *relevant* for practice decisions (Argyris, Putnam, and Smith 1985; Rapp and Poertner 1986; Rothman 1980; Weiss 1972: 119; Weissman 1977: 50). Hudson (1987:67) suggests that usable measures of service consumer problems must be "short, easy to read, easy to complete, easy to understand, easy to score, [and] easy to interpret . . ." Rapp (1984:78) suggests that performance reports should include a standard with which the performance can be compared.

Monitoring also requires skill in operationalization of indicators of program effort, efficiency, and effectiveness, and in the design of data-collection systems to implement service-evaluation programs. Intrinsic to effectiveness evaluation is the determination of *relative* standards for effectiveness. Particularly in programs for the severely disabled, program monitoring must establish realistic criteria for success. This can be done on the basis of norms achieved by existing programs (Carter 1987).

Operationalization of indicators to measure effort, efficiency, and effectiveness is feasible in the area of environmental practice because of its use of *concrete* services. Indicators for such services as employment, day care, housing, and training are more easily developed in comparison with counseling types of services, and lend themselves to the use of computers to store and retrieve data on the availability of these services.

The case study illustrates the use of monitoring for program efficiency and effectiveness. The CCMHC program evaluation design included *relative* measurements of program content as well as outcomes. Correlation of these two types of measures found that community resource coordination was a more efficient and effective technology than counseling.

Situational Influences

As in other skill areas, monitoring also requires the practitioner to appreciate the influence of situational factors. Lucas (1975) states that "the major reason most information systems have failed is that we have ignored organizational behavior problems in the design and operation of computer-based information systems" (6). Some of the organizational factors that have been identified are politics and power, resources, ideology, technology, decision making, and innovation and change (Weirich 1985).

Weissman (1987:206-207) cogently points to the effect of organizational context on an agency's ability to use service user feedback to further service effectiveness. The nature of the influence of the organizational context is tied to several unwarranted assumptions that link feedback to service effectiveness. One assumption is that there is agreement within organizations on goals and priorities. A second one is that rationality, rather than status and power, is the most influential factor determining organizational decisions. A third assumption is that organizations can transcend negative feedback. A fourth unwarranted assumption is that agency's are willing to change. A final assumption is that organizations are willing to accept the limitations on their autonomy that feedback can impose.

Given the above constraints, monitoring skill should include tactics and strategies for overcoming these barriers to the implementation of program evaluation. For example, the belief that monitoring the success or failure of staff effort is equivalent to professional suicide needs to be countered with evidence that indicates that, on the contrary, legitimacy and financial support can be enhanced through the use of accountability data (Rapp and Poertner 1987:34). Similarly, disagreement over organizational priorities, the role of status and power, and ambivalence toward change and limitations on autonomy needs to be considered in formulating an agenda for implementation of the monitoring system (Katz and Kahn 1978:675-679; Slavin 1985:313).

Another situational factor limiting the implementation of program evaluation are the misunderstandings that staff have regarding the monitoring of service consumer outcomes. Rapp and Poertner (1987) report on the following "myths" associated with outcome evaluations: outcomes are idiosyncratic; they cannot be measured; we cannot be held responsible for outcomes; and monitoring takes too much time and resources. Monitoring skill therefore includes the leadership skill needed to overcome the above sources of resistance to program evaluation.

Staff resistance to program monitoring stems in part from the inherent differences between program levels in their perception of criteria for service effectiveness and efficiency (Grasso and Epstein 1987:91). These different perceptions between lower- and upper-level staff leads to a "strain toward falsification" (Walker 1972).

One strategy for overcoming these situational barriers to successful monitoring is the active involvement of the practitioners in the design and development of the evaluation program (Weiner 1990:412-420). "Utilization oriented" evaluations should be geared to specific practice decisions and therefore will require staff input (Reid 1987:55). Staff are in a position to identify the "what," "who," and "why" of a monitoring system, which will help the monitor to determine the appropriate technology, or the "how" of the system (Slavin 1985:312).

Outcome-focused monitoring should obtain staff consensus as to the results that can realistically be expected. If this is achieved, then the staff can be given the autonomy to make decisions on the methods they will use to achieve these results. Allowing staff control over their activities facilitates their cooperation with a monitoring program.

Another strategy for motivating staff to participate in a monitoring system is making explicit how feedback of performance data relates to job requirements and organizational rewards. The explicit linking of rewards (e.g., merit raises, promotions, etc.) to work performance standards that are being monitored will increase the impact of feedback on the behavior of staff (Taylor 1987:191). A potential negative consequence could be staff falsification of the data in order to protect themselves. Monitoring skill requires the use of systematic checks to verify that the data collected is reliable and valid.

Monitoring programs that require consumer feedback need to recognize that service users may also be reluctant to cooperate. Service consumers are hesitant to criticize the services they receive for fear of punishment by service denial (Weissman 1987:209-210). This problem can be dealt with by assuring them of anonymity and by timing the feedback to occur at the termination of service (211).

As indicated above, feedback on the results of professional efforts can have a disrupting influence on the agency. Weissman (1987:214) suggests that the organization needs to have a method for obtaining "feedback on the feedback," as well as mechanisms for constructively dealing with the conflicts and tensions generated by making organizational performance visible. "Organizational ignorance is often functional in that it limits tension and limits dissent" (216). Weissman also cautions monitors to be alert to possible *dysfunctional* consequences ("social iatrogenisis") for staff and service consumers of program monitoring (209). Monitoring skills should therefore include methods for evaluating the effects of the monitoring program, both positive and negative. Furthermore, the organization has the responsibility to provide solutions to the problems revealed in the monitoring process, such as staff training or the addition of needed resources (Grasso and Epstein 1987; Williams 1975).

Since the monitoring of a system reveals the need for major or minor changes, skill is needed to plan for these different consequences (Weissman 1987:207-208). If the information revealed by monitoring points to the need for major system change, appropriate strategies should be used to implement the change (Neugeboren 1991:191,200).

The potential threat that monitoring poses to the system's power structure requires that this function be established close to the upper levels of authority and power (Kroeber and Watson 1979; Weirich

1985:317) and separated from line operations to prevent cooptation by the system. Accordingly, Weiss (1972:120-121) suggests that program evaluation functions be housed in planning and development units attached to the director's office.

Staff resistance to a monitoring system was evident in the case situation. Dr. Smith overcame this resistance by involving the direct practice staff in the formulation of the measures to be used to determine service outcomes. Also, the agency took the responsibility for retraining staff in community resource coordination techniques after the monitoring results revealed this to be an effective service intervention.

Leadership

Leadership skills *influence* others to maximize their contributions to program efforts (Simons 1985). Although leadership requires cognitive and affective abilities, it is also shaped by the situational factors. Different situational contexts have diverse leadership requirements. Leadership is used by environmental practitioners in performance of direct-service, as well as administration, social advocacy, planning, and policy formulation tasks.

Leadership Skills in Arenas of Practice

Micro level practitioners use leadership skills to influence staff in and outside their agencies to provide the resources needed by service users. This skill is used in community resource case coordination to influence service providers to coordinate services.

Macro level environmental practitioners use leadership skills to administer, plan, and implement policies. Direct-service agency administrators provide leadership at executive, middle management, and supervisory levels. The task of these administrators is to influence staff to participate actively in the accomplishment of agency objectives.

Community planners use leadership skills to accomplish better coordination and integration of human service programs. They use this skill to convince direct-service agency administrators of the benefits to be derived from cooperation and the cost of competition.

Leadership skills are also used to motivate agency administrators to modify dysfunctional programs and to experiment with new services. Social advocates use leadership skills in representing service consumer interests with administrators, planners, and policymakers.

Policy analysts use cognitive leadership skills to influence policymakers to modify dysfunctional policies and to develop new ones. Using their knowledge of the results of program efforts and the theoretical and empirical bases for experimenting with new initiatives, they exert their influence on policymakers to gain support for new programs.

The case situation illustrates the leadership role in the various arenas of practice. Ms. Jones, the direct-service practitioner, used influential skills to motivate the worker at the mental hospital to make more referrals. The line supervisors at CCMHC modified their leadership style in order to educate subordinates in environmental interventions. Dr. Smith used leadership skill to coordinate the Partial Care and Counseling departments. The planner, Mr. Wilson, successfully influenced the directors of CCMHC and the county mental hospital to improve coordination of their programs. The policy analyst used cognitive leadership in formulating a new mental health policy. The statewide citizens' committee use influential skills in advocating for the mentally ill.

Technical Aspects

The importance of any particular leadership skill will vary with the requirements of different levels of the organization. Upper-level leadership uses conceptual and policy-oriented skills, in contrast to lower-level direct practice and supervision, which employ affective skills. Upper-level "institutional" leadership is directed toward major system innovation. This skill uses both an *internal* and an *external* system perspective (Katz and Kahn 1978:540-543). An *external* perspective requires skill in assessment of environmental opportunities and demands. This is used to help the agency adapt to changes in the environment. The *internal* perspective helps in the coordination of internal agency operations.

Middle-level leadership facilitates the linkage between the upper and lower levels of the organization by bridging the interests and needs of these two levels. It also uses human relations skills to integrate staff and organizational goals (see the section on staffing below).

Lower-level supervisory skills motivate direct-service staff by setting clear and realistic expectations (Ehlers, Austin, and Prothero 1976:199-232). Supervisory leadership requires supportive and directive skills (Fleishman and Peters 1962:127-143). *Supportive* skill facilitates a nurturing work environment by "(a) creating a feeling of approval; (b) developing personal relations; (c) providing fair treatment; (d) enforcing rules equitably" (Austin 1981:301). *Directive* leadership structures subordinates' roles toward task accomplishment by providing technical support, in contrast to the social support given by supportive leadership.

Supportive leadership has been advocated as particularly appropriate for supervision in the human services. It is needed to moderate the stress induced by bureaucratic systems (Kadushin 1976). However, support in itself may not be enough to help the subordinate to cope with such systemic problems as high workload (Rauktis and Koeske 1994). Directive leadership can provide the technical help needed to work within dysfunctional systems.

The case situation illustrates the executive-level leadership skills of the policy analyst, the planner, and administrator in the creation of new policies for more and better services for the severely mentally ill. Dr. Smith practiced an external system perspective in the development of a public relations program to change the image of the agency. She also applied an internal system perspective in her coordination of two departments in the agency. The line supervisors modified their leadership skills from support to direction in order to train the workers in the new environmental interventions.

Situational Influences

As indicated above, direct-service administration leadership tasks vary with situational levels. Upper-level executives are responsible for maintaining an agency's public image in order to insure resource availability. Skills associated with the external system perspective are relevant for this task. In contrast, middle-level administrators need human relations leadership skills to integrate the staff into the organization. Lower-level leaders use technical case-related skills to supervise direct-service workers.

Situational influences are evident in the supervisory role within direct-service agencies. The effectiveness of either supportive or directive leadership depends on the nature of tasks to be performed (Hall 1977:244). Supportive supervision is effective when the work demands allow sufficient time for case decisions. In situations where time pressures are excessive, directive supervision is more appropriate.

Hersey and Blanchard's (1977) "situational leadership" model is a further example of the effect of the environment on leadership. This model relates supervisory behavior with the nature of the task to be performed and the competence of the supervisee. Four different roles are employed in this model, varying by degree of supervisory support and direction. These roles are telling, selling, participating, and delegating, and the appropriateness of any role is dependent on the level of competence of the subordinate. As the level of competence of supervisee improves, supervisory leadership moves from telling to delegating.

Situational influences on lower leadership were evident in the case situation. Demands on line workers to perform a different type of intervention required directive rather than supportive supervision. The differential leadership skills associated with various organizational levels were evident in the leadership deficits in middle management. Their responsibility for integration of staff abilities and organizational needs was not fulfilled, since they were hiring personnel who were not trained to serve the severely mentally ill. The upper-level leadership skill was demonstrated by the director's efforts to change the public image of the agency.

Staffing

The overall objective of staffing is the *integration of individual staff and system goals.* Staffing activities include staff recruitment, selection, training, and performance appraisal (Austin, M. J. 1981:157-280; Ehlers, Austin, and Prothero 1976:161-198; Lewis and Lewis 1983: 98-116).

Human service agencies are labor intensive organizations. Given the significant part played by staff in the achievement of agency goals, staffing skills can be crucial to program effectiveness.

Staffing in Arenas of Practice

Staffing skills are used on both the micro and macro levels of environmental practice. In the direct-service context, it is important for the worker to have a clear understanding of how his/her individual skills, interests, and goals can be integrated with job requirements. This occurs first in the staff recruitment and selection process when the direct-service worker seeks a position that meets his/her individual interests, skills, and career goals. For example, while searching for employment and being interviewed for a position, a direct-service worker will need to evaluate official job descriptions, obtain information about the agency's philosophy, and become familiar with the specific expectations associated with the job. If the person lacks the required skills, the opportunity for in-service training should be explored during the job application process.

Direct-service workers have also been used to help recruit appropriate staff for vacant positions. Particularly in the field of environmental practice, where there are relatively few persons with the philosophical interest or skill necessary to achieve environmental change, direct-service staff can help to recruit via their personal networks. It is in the self-interest of direct-service staff to help recruit staff who have similar professional interests, as this will help facilitate harmonious working relationships.

Staffing skills are also important for human service professionals working in administration, planning, and policy. Administrators of direct-service agencies need staffing skills to carry out the personnel management functions of recruitment, selection, training, and performance appraisal. These functions are not only important for system maintenance, but also are essential for the accomplishment of organizational change, which depends on finding staff with skills different from those possessed by staff that the organization had previously hired.

Community planners need staffing skills to help direct-service agencies in their recruitment of environmentally oriented practitioners. This role is appropriate for planners who are attempting to facilitate the innovation of environmental programs which require different kinds of staff. Policy analysts also use staffing skills to help shape personnel policies and procedures for funding environmentally focused programs.

In the case situation, Dr. Smith used staffing skills in the development of new policies for recruitment, selection, training, and performance evaluation. The policy analyst and community planner also used staffing skills in the formulation of a new educational program for training professionals for service to the mentally disabled.

Technical Aspects

Staffing first requires the design of organization roles and expectations, which are translated into written job descriptions. This is done in order to assure that staff recruitment, selection, training, and performance appraisal are done in conformity with these previously designed roles (Neugeboren 1991:60).

Recruitment should be targeted toward sources that can be expected to provide persons whose philosophy and skills are congruent with environmental practice goals. Since most human-service training is geared to individual-change models, recruitment of environmentally oriented practitioners will need to be selective. For direct-service staff, a good source for environmentally oriented practitioners would be undergraduate social work programs that have field training in public sector agencies serving the severely disabled. Undergraduates majoring in environmental and community psychology, political science, sociology, and economics can be expected to have a macro orientation and would be additional sources for recruitment. Master's level social workers educated in the community organization area are another potential source. Macro level environmentally oriented practitioners can be recruited from educational programs in administration, planning, and policy in schools of social work, public health, and urban planning.

Selection procedures are used to determine if individuals recruited have the philosophy and skills congruent with environmental practice. The interview as a selection device can have serious shortcomings because of its tendency to overemphasize the interpersonal skills of the applicant. Traditional testing procedures as used in civil service selection also have not been validated with practice skills (Steiner 1977:39). Selection approaches have therefore turned more to procedures and that simulate practice situations (Lewis and Lewis

1983:105). The "assessment center" model for staff selection and development emphasizes the use of simulation exercises (McGee and Crow 1982:12). The U.S. government has instituted a system for use of college grade point average and skills tests as a selection procedure for federal civil service positions. Entrance tests for more than 100 jobs have been eliminated since 1982 after it was found that the Professional and Administrative Career Examination was racially discriminatory (*The New York Times* 1988).

In-service *training* is another mechanism used to integrate staff skills with organizational needs. Training can focus on three areas: (1) improving task accomplishment in the immediate job; (2) prepareing for individual career mobility; and (3) preparing the individual for development within the organization.

Training for practice should be oriented toward applications and skills. Experiential types of training, which use techniques such as gaming or simulations, are appropriate for instructing in practice skills and tasks (McGee and Crow 1982:14-15).

Objective staff *performance appraisal* is critical for agency effectiveness. Performance-appraisal data is used in feedback to the practitioner to guide corrective action. Fair organizational reward and sanction procedures are dependent on objective staff performance appraisals. The design of appropriate employee training and placement programs also require a systematic performance appraisal system (Sauser 1980:13).

Performance appraisals can focus on employee efforts and/or results. Ratings can be done of attitudes and/or behavior. A desirable appraisal system evaluates behaviors that distinguish between successful and unsuccessful job performance (Lewis and Lewis 1983:107). A system that links performance with service user benefit is most desirable, but rarely is used (Nurius and Hudson 1988: 359; Wiehe 1980:6-7).

Different appraisal procedures consist of behavioral-anchored rating scales, job-related skills tests, and critical-incident techniques (Lewis and Lewis 1983:108-109). Since absolute measures of performance are difficult to achieve in human service practice, performance appraisal is done on a comparison basis. Staff are ranked in relationship to colleagues who have similar tasks.

Staffing skills were used in the case situation. Dr. Smith used these skills to recruit persons with training in community organization for direct-service positions. Simulation tests geared to environmental manipulation intervention skills were instituted. In-service training for administrative and direct-service staff was also established. A merit award system was established that was linked with the staff performance of environmental practice skills.

Situational Influences on Staffing

Staffing activities can be influenced by organizational contextual factors. For example, in-service training, if established in separate staff development units, can become divorced from the realities of practice. When this occurs, staff will resist cooperation (Reid and Beard 1980:81). Trainers need communication links with practitioners to insure that they are fully aware of the skills required.

The value of staff performance appraisal systems are perceived differently at various levels. Supervisors believe more strongly than workers that performance standards are an effective means of evaluating work performance (Harkness and Mulinski 1988:342). This relates to supervisory responsibility for performance evaluations. The different perceptions of the value of performance appraisal systems should be taken into account in the planning and implementation of this kind of a system.

Although objective and performance evaluations are the desired goal, situational factors can result in arbitrary and capricious reward systems. For example, in situations where new administrators assume office, the principle of a "new broom sweeps clean" may operate (i.e., to insure loyalty), new administrators may use arbitrary and biased performance criteria to remove those who were hired under the previous management. This is illustrated in a situation where an incoming manager, offended by a party given for the administrator who was being replaced, used this as a reason to fire the person who arranged the event.

Staff participation in other activities such as recruitment and selection will also be influenced by their roles and service philosophies. Thus, existing staff might be reluctant to recruit and select staff who are unusually competent for fear that they will not be able to compete successfully with them for agency rewards. Similarly, they will be hesitant to recruit and select staff whose professional ideologies they cannot accept. This will make it difficult to recruit environmentally oriented staff into an agency where the personnel find this orientation in conflict with their individual-focused philosophy.

The case situation illustrates how the clinical environment of the CCMHC constrained the selection and recruitment of environmentally oriented staff. The power struggle between the clinically and environmentally oriented staff was dealt with by the director's creation of a community resource coordination unit that had its own power base. She also removed the hiring function from the middle managers, who also were constraining the selection of environmentally oriented staff. Environmental constraints were also present at the School of Social Work, which also was dominated by clinically oriented faculty.

Negotiating

Negotiation is a process through which parties come to agreements. Negotiating occurs between interdependent individuals and organizations, and is used in competitive as well as cooperative situations. The goal of negoation is to obtain agreements among departments, both within organizations and between agencies, to resolve conflicts and coordinate and integrate efforts. Negotiating skills create consensus by stressing complementary interests derived from shared goals and resource exchange (Holloway and Brager 1985; Neugeboren 1991: 216-218; Popple 1984). As with the skill areas previously discussed, negotiating outcomes depend not only on individual practitioner abilities but also on environmental factors (Lauffer 1984:116).

Negotiating in Arenas of Practice

Micro and macro environmental practitioners use negotiating skills to integrate assistance for service users. At the micro level, the case coordinator applies negotiating skills to obtain resources for service consumers from other agencies. Direct-service practitioners develop exchange relationships with workers within their own agencies and staff in other agencies to negotiate case-coordination agreements for jointly served service users.

The case illustrates the use of negotiating skills by the direct-service worker at the CCMHC. Ms. Jones used these skills to develop an agreement with the worker at the county mental hospital to obtain predischarge information on jointly served service consumers.

At the macro level, environmental practitioners use negotiating skills in direct-service agency administration, community planning, and policy formulation. Direct-service agency administrators apply negotiating skills to coordinate departments within their organizations. These skills focus on integrating the objectives of subunits by stressing shared organizational goals. Administrators use authority and power to influence the development of cooperative relations between departmental units. Direct-service agency administrators also use negotiating skills to link their agencies with other community programs through the development of affiliation agreements. These negotiated agreements use common goals and resource exchange as the basis for explicating the need for cooperative relations between agencies. Negotiating skills are used to overcome such barriers to inter-agency cooperation as turf protectiveness and fear of loss of autonomy (Lauffer 1984:96-116).

The use of negotiating skills in direct-service administration is illustrated in the case situation where Dr. Smith facilitated coordination between the Partial Care and Counseling departments of the CCMHC. She used her position of authority to persuade the two department heads to cooperate in working toward their common goal of service user aid. Negotiating skills use shared goals of service user benefit as a motivating force to achieve cooperation.

Community planners use negotiating skills to promote interagency coordination. Community planners act as mediators and arbitrators in negotiating interagency conflict (Lauffer 1984:113). They obtain interorganizational cooperation by making agencies aware of their shared goals and opportunities for resource exchange. Community planners use their authority derived from their allocation of funds to influence agencies to negotiate affiliation agreements. Policy analysts use negotiating skills in their work with policymakers to develop environmental programs that will enhance service consumer benefit. Negotiating focuses on the common interests of the different interests groups to obtain policy consensus.

In the case situation, Dr. Wilson, the community planner, served as a mediator between the CCMHC and the county mental hospital and helped produce in an interagency agreement to hold joint case conferences on patients being discharged into the community. The policy analyst used negotiating skills to influence the School of Social Work to develop a special training program for persons working with the severely mentally ill.

Technical Aspects

The technical aspects of negotiating are categorized as *types, stages, strategies, and tactics* (Popple 1984), and the skills needed to promote an *exchange process.*

Types of Negotiation Processes. The different types of negotiation processes are distributive bargaining, and integrative bargaining, attitudinal structuring, intraorganizational bargaining, mediation and arbitration. *Distributive bargaining* is a competitive or "win-lose" approach to negotiations, in contrast to *integrative bargaining* which is a "win-win" cooperative approach that results in gain to both parties (Lauffer 1984:99-100). The exchange framework discussed below assumes an integrative approach to negotiation. It provides a basis for turning "win-lose" predicaments into "win-win" opportunities (Lauffer 1984:111-112). In the case situation, an integrative bargaining approach was used in the negotiation of the agreement between Ms. Jones and Ms. Williams.

Attitudinal structuring involves the manipulation of the opponent's attitudes. Examples of attitudinal structuring are "demand creation"–building up the perceived value of the commodity being offered. The opposite–"motivational withdrawal"–occurs when the buyer convinces the seller that he/she has less interest in the commodity under consideration (Tedeschi and Rosenfeld 1980). *Intraorganizational bargaining* involves negotiating within one's own organization to resolve any disagreements that would prevent a united front at the negotiating table. In the case example, Ms. Jones and Ms. Williams conducted intraorganizational bargaining with their respective supervisors to insure support for the final negotiated agreement.

Mediation and *arbitration* are procedures in which a third party intervenes to facilitate the negotiating process. Arbitration often is compulsory in that it involves the advance agreement of the parties that recommendations proposed are binding. In contrast, mediation is voluntary, with nonbinding recommendations (Lauffer 1984:112-113). In the case, Dr. Wilson, the planner, served as mediator between the CCMHC and the county mental hospital.

Stages of Negotiating. Negotiation involves preconference, conference, and postconference stages (Karrass 1970). Different types of bargaining are appropriate for these three stages.

The *preconference* stage uses integrative bargaining to obtain agreement that it is in the self-interest of the parties to engage in serious deliberations. Attitude structuring is also used at this stage to set the tone for the negotiations in terms of an overall strategy (e.g., make the opponent see them as tough, indispensable, cooperative, etc.). Intraorganizational bargaining is used in the preconference stage of negotiation in order to establish a united front at the bargaining table.

The preconference stage was illustrated in the case situation where Ms. Jones and Ms. Williams initially agreed to their common goals of service to the severely mentally ill. They also agreed that there was a joint need for a better method for exchange of information on jointly served patients. A preconference meeting was also held between Ms. Jones and her supervisor to obtain agreement on the strategy and tactics to be used at the forthcoming meeting.

The *conference* stage involves three phases: establishing the negotiating range; reconnoitering the negotiating range; and precipitating the decision- making crisis (Douglas 1962). It is during this stage that the parties hammer out an agreement.

During the first conference phase, *establishing the negotiating range,* the parties explore the potential "stretch of territory" within which the parties are willing to negotiate. In this stage, the parties state impossible demands to test the outer limits of the range within which they will reach an agreement. This phase uses intraorganizational bargaining to obtain internal consensus on where to set outer limits, and attitudinal structuring to impress the opposition with their conviction.

In the second conference phase, *reconnoitering the negotiating range,* distributive bargaining predominates. During this phase, there is shift from promoting one's own position to attacking the opponent's in order to gain some idea of what the other party will concede.

The third conference stage, *precipitating the decision-making process,* concludes either with a formal agreement or an impasse. Intraorganizational bargaining is increased in order to obtain clearance of the final offers.

In the case situation, Ms. Jones established the negotiation range by making the extreme demand for participation in hospital case conferences. This precipitated an impasse which required an adjournment of the negotiating sessions in order for each worker to confer with their respective supervisors. At a second meeting, an agreement was reached on the lesser demand for a two-week notification procedure of pending discharges from the hospital to the CCMHC.

The *postconference stage* uses integrative bargaining to formalize and implement the agreement. It involves agreement elaboration, approval, administration, and closure (Karrass 1970). In the case situation, the postconference meeting was held to work out the details of the agreement for the two-week notification procedure, including the kinds of information that would be provided by the hospital to the CCMHC.

Strategies and Tactics of Negotiation. Strategies refers to the overall plans for a negotiation, while tactics are the maneuvers employed to implement the strategy. Strategies and tactics vary depending on the stage of negotiation.

In the preconference stage, the goal is to develop an overall negotiation strategy. The following tactics are used in this stage:

- *List Issues*–Issues are listed as problems rather than as demands in order to allow for more than one solution.
- *Study the Opposition*–Obtain as much information as possible about the opposition, including the relevant policies of the opponent's agency.
- *Analyze Your Own Position*–Assess the strengths and weaknesses of your position.
- *Formulate Goals*–Formulate goals based on issues listed and an analysis of your opponent's and your own positions. Goals are categorized in terms of those that are essential, desirable, and tradable (Hermone 1974).

- *Develop an Agenda*–Taking the initiative of presenting an agenda has the advantage of defining issues on your terms. The disadvantage is that it reveals your position in advance and gives the opposition an opportunity to prepare a rebuttal.
- *Decide on Negotiation Site*–Meeting at your own site has the advantage of having access to others for consultation. Going to your opponent's location enables you to interrupt negotiations on the ground that approval is needed by higher authorities.

In the case, various strategies and tactics were used by Ms. Jones in the preconference stage of negotiations. The basic *issue* agreed upon with the supervisor was that a better referral procedure was needed for patients discharged from the mental hospital. A *study of the opposition* determined that the hospital would be reluctant to allow Ms. Jones to participate in their meetings. An *analysis of the CCMHC's position* determined that their strength was the pressure for better coordination coming from the county and state levels. A weakness in their position was their lack of authority to make demands on the county mental hospital.

A *formulation of goals* by Ms. Jones and her supervisor determined that it was essential to obtain *early* notification of the discharge of patients. Participation in hospital meetings, while desirable,was not essential and therefore could be traded for an agreement to two week's prior notification of patient discharge. The use of the hospital as a *negotiation site* provided Ms. Jones with an excuse for interrupting the negotiations to consult with her supervisor.

It is at the conference stage that strategies and tactics are most evident. The following are some of the strategies and tactics that can be used in this stage.

- *Seating Arrangement*–Sitting at the head of the table has the advantage of placing a person in a position of authority. Separating your opponents at the negotiating table decreases their ability to join together in opposition.
- *Opening the Meeting*–Taking the initiative to open the meeting allows you to control the discussion. Starting by reviewing ground rules can prevent later misunderstandings.
- *Concession Behavior*–Successful negotiators avoid making first concessions, concede slowly, and avoided making con-

cessions as large as those of their opponents (Karrass 1970). A general principle is to only give something away if some concession is given in return.

- *Aspiration Level*–Negotiators with a high level of aspirations obtain better settlements. A general principle is to develop aspiration level on the basis of the cost of the breakdown of the negotiations.
- *Revealing Your Position*–Revealing your position too early may lead your opposition to press for additional concessions. Waiting too long to reveal your position risks appearing inflexible.
- *Authority*–Always be clear as to whether the person you are negotiating with has the authority to make decisions. If that person does not have authority, you will have to plan accordingly.

In the case situation, Ms. Williams did not have *authority* to allow Ms. Jones to participate in hospital meetings. This contingency was planned for by allowing time for consultation with supervisors. Ms. Jones took the initiative to *open the meeting* and *revealed her position* first. She continued to show *high aspirations* by demanding participation in hospital staff meetings. However, she was careful not to reveal her "bottom line" demand of a two-week notification procedure until the latter part of the negotiation process. Ms. Jones structured the negotiation process so that Ms. Williams made the first concession. Her counter offer of a four-week prior notification procedure enabled a final agreement that achieved her negotiation goal of a two-week prior notification procedure.

In the postconference stage, an integrative strategy is most appropriate. Cooperation is stressed in order to maximize implementation of the agreement. In the case, a follow-up meeting worked out the details of the agreement, including the specific kinds of information that would be needed by the CCMHC to carry out the aftercare of patients discharged from the hospital.

Exchange Skills. Negotiation uses an *exchange* framework to promote inter- and intraorganizational cooperation. It necessitates an understanding of how inter- and intraorganizational competition can be mediated and cooperation can be facilitated through the voluntary exchange of complementary resources to achieve shared goals (Reid 1965:359).

The first task of the negotiator in implementing the exchange process is to highlight *shared goals.* The negotiator has to be aware that goal *perception* by different parties is just as important as whether the goals are in reality commonly held. In addressing the task of highlighting shared goals, the negotiator has to also understand the impact that official as opposed to operative goals will have on the negotiating process. As *official* goals are the basis for agency legitimation and support, they are instrumental for the *initiation* of cooperative efforts. *Implementation* of the exchange will be influenced by the extent to which *operative* goals are shared (Neugeboren 1991:216). Negotiating requires not only making opponents aware of goal similarity, but also showing how the goals of one unit can facilitate the goal accomplishment of another unit.

Achievement of complementary goals is done through *resource exchange.* The opportunity for an exchange of resources such as personnel, information, funds, legitimation, equipment, and office quarters provides the impetus for cooperative behavior. Negotiating skill overcomes political, economic, and psychological barriers to cooperation between interdependent parties by highlighting these opportunities for the exchange of complementary resources.

In the case situation, the inadequate coordination between the Partial Care and Counseling departments at the CCMHC was due to the perception of the department chiefs that these two units did not share common goals. After Dr. Smith convinced the department chiefs that the goals were complementary, efforts to cooperate through an exchange of scarce resources of office space could proceed.

The lack of coordination between the CCMHC and the county mental hospital was due in part to the discrepancy between the official and operative goals of the hospital. Although the official goals of the hospital stressed the value of community care, the operative goals of some of the staff favored in-patient care. The fact that the official goals of these two agencies were compatible enabled Ms. Jones and Ms. Williams to *initiate* a discussion of ways that referrals could be expedited. Since Ms. Jones was aware that some of the professionals at the hospital did not favor community care, she had to be selective in approaching a social worker who favored community care.

The potential for a cooperative relationship between the direct-service workers at the CCMHC and the county hospital was enhanced by their awareness of the potential for resource exchange. The exchange of information resources was seen as mutually beneficial to both parties.

Situational Influences

The results of negotiations are influenced as much by external factors as by the skill of the individual negotiator. For example, the influence of power on the negotiating process should be taken into account (Lauffer 1984:34-36). Power is the capacity to obtain involuntary compliance. Since the achievement of consensus in any negotiating process assumes voluntary agreement, it requires equality in power. But the distribution of power varies from one situation to the next, so it behooves the negotiator to do a prior assessment of the power conditions before engaging in the negotiation process.

The exchange model for negotiation skills assumes that the parties involved clearly recognize their self-interest. However, there often are situations where disagreements are related to symbolic and ideological differences (Lauffer 1984:101; Neugeboren 1991: 230). Ideological conflicts cannot be successfully negotiated since they are based on strongly held beliefs that cannot be compromised. Environmental practitioners need to be aware of the potential for ideological conflicts related to philosophical differences as to the cause and solution of service user problems: the person vs. the environment. A strategy for avoiding ideological conflicts is to focus the discussions on concrete substantive and procedural issues (Lauffer 1984:100-101). In the case situation, Dr. Smith avoided becoming involved in the philosophical differences of the chiefs of the Counseling and Partial Care departments by focussing on the advantages of sharing resources (office quarters).

Negotiating within an intraorganizational context to achieve coordination of different departments also requires an appreciation of the situational influences of organizational subsystems. The managerial task of coordinating different subunits in an agency necessitates an understanding of subsystem functions, dynamics, and mechanisms (Neugeboren 1991:69-88). The theory underlying this organic model of organizations assumes that there are five subsystems that have different purposes, philosophies, and tasks that need to be coordinated and integrated (Hasenfeld 1983:44). The direct-service agency administrator uses this knowledge of subsystems to negotiate conflicts arising between departments and successfully integrate their efforts towards the shared goal of service consumer benefit. This was demonstrated in the case, where Dr. Smith facilitated coordination between the Partial Care and Counseling departments.

Representing

Representing requires skills in public relations and marketing. Its purpose is to gain public understanding, acceptance, and support by articulating agency policies and programs to various constituency groups, including consumers, resource providers, community leaders and other service agencies (Ehlers, Austin, and Prothero 1976:271; Schneider and Sharon 1982:60). Situational factors also influence this skill area (e.g., representation to constituency groups requires an understanding of the interdependency between the agency and these external groups).

Representing in Arenas of Practice

Representing skills are used in micro and macro environmental practice. Direct-service practitioners use representing skills in interpreting programs to service users and other agencies (Schmidt and Weiner 1966:78-82). In advocating for the service consumer, the direct-service case worker represents the service user's interests to agencies to whom referral is made (see Chapter 4). The micro practitioner also is responsible for acquainting staff in other human service agencies with policies and procedures affecting case decision making. The general purpose of representing on the direct-service level is to develop and maintain a positive public image with staff from agencies with whom there are ongoing working relationships. Representatives also serve this purpose when disseminate information on agency programs by speaking before public groups.

In the case situation, Ms. Jones performed a representing function in her contacts with Ms. Williams at the county mental hospital.

Administrators of direct-service agencies use representing skills to obtain legitimacy and community support from groups external to the agency (Schmidt and Weiner 1966:45-64). Public relations programs are used to enhance the potential for obtaining resources for the agency by developing a positive public image. Representing skills are also used by agency administrators in the development of inter-agency collaboration. Affiliation agreements with other community agencies are achieved by demonstrating the extent to which agency goals and purposes are congruent with those of other community programs. In the case, Dr. Smith used representing skills in developing a public relations program to enhance the community's image of the CCMHC.

Community planners use representing skills to explain their role and responsibilities in planning and coordinating services. Their allocation and monitoring of funds to service providers requires skill in interpreting the responsibility of the planning agency in facilitating a more efficient and effective community network of services. Policy analysts use representing skills to help planners and service providers appreciate the goals of policy formulators who have promulgated statutes and policies. In the case situation, Mr. Wilson, the community planner, used representing skills to facilitate coordination between the CCMHC and the county mental hospital. The policy analyst also used these kinds of skills in promoting a special education program at the School of Social Work for training BSW and MSW students in the skills needed to serve the severely disabled.

Technical Aspects

Representing consists of three elements: evaluation, action, and communication (Ehlers, Austin, and Prothero 1976:271). Public relations, which is intrinsic to representing, has been defined as "the management function which evaluates public attitudes, identifies the policies and procedures of an organization with the public interest, and executes a program of action and communication to reach public understanding and acceptance" (Marston 1963:5).

Evaluation of public opinion determines the positive and negative attitudes of the constituency groups on which the agency is dependent (Katz and Kahn 1978:139-140). Information can be obtained from agency staff who have contact with the public. Media presentations on the agency's programs can also be used as indicators of public attitudes toward the agency. The process of evaluating public opinion may reveal unmet service needs that can lead to the development of new "products" (Lauffer 1986:39).

The identification of the organization's policies with the public interest links the evaluation of public opinion with agency goals and purposes. A program of *action* consists of the use of communication devices to influence the public to identify with the agency's goals (Ehlers, Austin, and Prothero 1976:274).

In the case situation, the Department of Mental Health used representing skills to evaluate the public's attitudes toward the lack of adequate community programs for the mentally ill homeless. This led to the identification of the need for a new policy initiative which established a program for action requiring the community mental health centers to establish programs for the severely mentally ill. The department informed the public of the new policy for community care of the mentally ill through public meetings, which were used as a device for enlisting community support for this program.

Marketing and representing are interrelated activities. Marketing focuses on the needs of key groups such as consumers, resource suppliers and other service providers to determine how available services accommodate their needs (Lauffer 1986:32). The goal of marketing is to determine which markets should be targeted for penetration. Representing skills are used to inform relevant groups of the services that can meet their needs. Therefore, representing is a tool used in the marketing of human service programs.

The tools of representing include media publicity (Schmidt and Weiner 1966:184-217), periodicals, brochures, public speaking, conferences, personal communications, and special events (Ehlers, Austin, and Prothero 1976:272-273). The press release is a basic tool used in representing (Ehlers, Austin, and Prothero 275-279). A study of the effectiveness of marketing revealed that face-to-face approaches are most successful and the use of media is least effective (Kaye 1994). In the case situation, the community planner used a public meeting covered by the press to obtain publicity about the need for better program coordination.

Responsibility for representing resides within the executive level of agencies (Brown 1966:47-48). Centralized control of this activity is necessary in order to insure that representation efforts are coordinated in a manner that insures that agency credibility is established and maintained. In order to achieve a positive public image, representation activities should be ongoing (Schmidt and Weiner 1966:28-44), rather than an ad-hoc response to specific crises (Schneider and Sharon 1982:61).

Agency board members play an instrumental role in helping the executive obtain legitimacy, community acceptance, and support (Schmidt and Weiner 1966:83-98). Participation of the board's consumer representatives can enhance the legitimacy of the agency in the eyes of consumers and facilitate recruitment of service users into the program. Different approaches are used when initially attempting to achieve community legitimation and support than are used to insure the ongoing maintenance of that support.

In the *initiation* phase, the executive selects board members who have the status to influence community image makers, such as the media and key community leaders. Board members are also chosen based on their ability to influence the agency's constituency groups of consumers and other service providers. In this phase, the board members are educated about the agency's goals and purposes, how the programs are intended to achieve these ends, and the various public relations problems that can be expected to occur. Training board members to anticipate various community pressures on the agency can facilitate their role as community buffer and interpreter when problems do occur. This is necessary especially for human service programs that serve socially deviant service user groups that the community will pressure the agency to control.

Maintenance of agency legitimacy and community acceptance requires an ongoing public relations program. These representation efforts are directed at the general public, as well as at other agencies in the community. They employ various methods for communicating to external groups, including the media (Brawley 1985). Ongoing interpretation of program efforts and successes through newsletters, brochures, press releases, and shows participation on radio and television helps to insure that a positive public image will be maintained. Representation of an agency's program also occurs on an individual basis through exposure of influential community members to the agency's program activities. This allows them to personally observe service consumers' problem situations and agency intervention. In a field such as environmental practice, it is particularly important to educate community leaders about the unique value of this kind of intervention compared with the more traditional people-changing programs.

The case situation illustrates representing in the responsibility taken by the director of the CCMHC in initiating an ongoing public relations program to change the negative public image of the agency. Board members were recruited who could convey to the community the problems associated with housing and employment of the mentally ill.

Since representing has the purpose of *selling* and marketing agency programs, it requires an understanding of the values and interests of the different constituency groups. The general publics' attitudes toward social problems, both positive and negative, must be understood in order to "package" the specific program in terms that are acceptable to relevant groups. Representing will be enhanced if agency goals are linked with established public values, such as individual independence and self-sufficiency, upward mobility, and support for dependent persons such as children and the disabled. This is illustrated in the case situation where the Department of Mental Health used the public's discontent with the mentally ill homeless who were living in the streets to initiate the new policy of community care for this group.

Promoting a program with other service providers requires an understanding of whether their programs complement or compete with those of the agency. If competition is the dominant mode, then strategies must be devised to emphasize the potential for cooperation. Marketing a program with sponsors and funding authorities also requires an understanding of their priorities and goals.

Representing is heavily dependent on communication skills. This includes presenting information simply and clearly including use of visual aids to highlight the message to be delivered. Skills in graphics, videotape preparation, and verbal and written communication are useful in representation activities. In the case situation, the planner used various representing devices to enlist public support for a program of better coordination of services for the mentally ill, including the press, television, and the influence of a local politician.

Situational Influences

Situational aspects of representing arise from the dependency between the agency and the constituent groups to whom it needs to market its programs. The particular nature of the dependency on resource suppliers, consumers, provider agencies, or community leaders will determine which representing activities are appropriate.

Representing activities with sponsors and funding authorities require prior knowledge of the particular interests and goals of these organizations. Foundations and government planning and allocating agencies have specific mandates to guide the assignment of funds. Requests for proposals (RFPs) disclose the "official" criteria for fund allocation. There are, however, unofficial or hidden criteria that also influence decisions of the funding authorities. Representing efforts to obtain these funds must take into account both official and unofficial criteria. Unofficial criteria can be ascertained by personal contact with staff who can provide this "inside" information.

Representing with other service providers also requires an understanding of the interdependency with these agencies (Schmidt and Weiner 1966:129-137). Knowledge of shared goals and the potential for resource exchange aids in the development of marketing strategies to convince these agencies of the value of developing an exchange relationship. The mode and content of representing activities will be influenced by the specific opportunities for the sharing of resources.

Representing activities with such influential community members as politicians, community leaders, and the media also require an appreciation of their agendas. A politician's need for public visibility can be used by an agency to obtain legitimation and community support. The same is true with regard to other community leaders. Representatives can also exploit the media's need for newsworthy stories that will increase their audience. Representatives use their understanding of these interests in order that will develop public relations packages that will enlist the support of these organizations.

In the case situation, the Department of Mental Health used the public concern about the homeless to promote the program of community care for the mentally ill. The community planner involved a politician to help promote better coordination of mental health programs.

INTERRELATIONSHIP BETWEEN SKILL AREAS

It is evident that in practice situations the above skills are interrelated. However, the cognitive decision-making skill would naturally precede the more action-oriented skills such as negotiating or leadership. Thus, the assessment process of determining negotiating strategies requires problem definition and evaluation of alternative solutions prior to actually entering into negotiations.

The influence process contained in use of leadership skills naturally occurs in tandem with such other skill areas as representing, staffing, negotiating, and monitoring. Promotional efforts in representing use referent and expert power to maintain constituency support. Leadership skills are also needed to influence staff to overcome their resistance to program monitoring.

Training skills which are used in staffing are related to monitoring efforts if it is determined that program deficiencies are the result of to undertrained employees. Program marketing (representing) is dependent on the exchange process, which is also the basis for negotiating.

The skills discussed above are summarized in the following chart, which links each skill with its objectives. The key word(s) which describes each skill is underlined.

Skill	Purpose
Decision Making	*Problem Solving*–analyze cause and determine objectives
Monitoring	*Verify* achievement of objectives
Leadership	*Influence* behavior
Negotiating	Consensus via *shared interests*
Staffing	*Integrate* individual and system goals
Representing	*Promote* agency programs

SUMMARY

This chapter discussed six skills that are used in environmental practice: decision making, monitoring, leadership, staffing, negotiating, and representing. The case example was used to illustrate the use of these skills in a practice situation. The discussion highlighted both the technical and the political character of practice skills, as well as the commonality of micro and macro practice skills.

The six skill areas were discussed in terms of four arenas of practice: direct practice, administration of direct-service agencies, community planning, and policy analysis. The technical aspects of each skill area were presented along with the situational influences that affect the practical application of the various skills. Finally, the interdependence of these six skills in practice was also reviewed.

STUDY QUESTIONS

1. Select a situation where you had to make a decision in your work in a human service agency. Discuss how situational factors affected your efforts to be "rational" in making the decision.

2. You have been given responsibility for implementing a program evaluation system in an agency where you work. What skills would you use to insure the cooperation of staff in the implementation of this system?

3. You are supervising a new worker who is unfamiliar with the requirements of her job. She reacts negatively to your direction. What skills would you use to deal with this situation?

4. You have been given responsibility for developing a system for recruiting, selecting, training, and evaluating staff to insure their competence in environmental practice. Discuss what steps you would take to accomplish this task.

5. You are the director of the CCMHC and want to negotiate an affiliation agreement with the county mental hospital for a joint program of community care for the severely mentally ill. Discuss what strategies and tactics you would use to develop this agreement.

6. You are an administrator of a child welfare agency that has received criticism in the media following the death of a child under its care. Discuss a public relations program that you would institute to enhance the public image of your agency.

Chapter 4

COMMUNITY RESOURCE COORDINATION ON THE MICRO LEVEL

Community Resource Coordination on the Micro Level

INTRODUCTION

This chapter discusses community resource coordination with specific emphasis on the micro, or case, level of intervention. Macro resource coordination, which involves the roles of the direct service agency administrator, the community planner, and the policy analyst will be covered in the next chapter. Although the micro and macro levels of community resource coordination are treated separately, it is an assumption of the conceptual framework of this book that they are interrelated and that effective intervention on each of these levels requires knowledge of both levels. Thus, the case coordinator needs to understand that the macro practitioner performs tasks that provide necessary support for micro intervention. Similarly, the administrator, planner, and policy analyst need to appreciate the roles and tasks performed by the case coordinator in order to fulfill those supportive functions.

Community resource coordination focuses on creating linkages between formal organizations. The linking of service users with informal support networks will be dealt with in the chapters on social support (Chapters 5 and 6).

This chapter begins with a case example that will be referred to throughout this and the next chapter in order to illustrate the principles and practices of community resource coordination. The intervention skills of decision making, negotiating, and representing are also linked in this chapter with the activities of the community resource case coordinator. (See Chapter 3 for a detailed discussion of practice skills.)

CASE: CASE COORDINATION IN A FAMILY SERVICE AGENCY

Betty Jones is a service consumer of the Central County family social services. She was recently discharged from the county mental hospital with a diagnosis of schizophrenia. She had ten previous admissions to this hospital. Upon release to the community, the hospital discharge planner recommended the following services: housing, financial aid, vocational training, and psychiatric treatment. She was referred for service by the hospital to the family social service agency (FSSA) under a recently instituted joint program with the county mental hospital. An agreement was signed by these two agencies whereby all patients discharged into the community served by the social service agency will receive case coordination service from the FSSA.

The caseworker at the FSSA referred Betty to the community mental health center (CMHC) for psychiatric treatment, but was unsuccessful because Betty failed to follow through on appointments. The CMHC staff concluded that she was not suitable for their service because she was not "motivated" for help. Betty was dissatisfied with the psychological focus of the service offered by the CMHC, since she perceived her main problems to be the lack of a job and a place to live. She was particularly interested in doing word processing. She also wanted to live in her own apartment although she did not have sufficient funds to pay rent.

This case was not unique. The caseworkers at the FSSA had repeated difficulties obtaining mental health services for their service users, who had severe disabilities, because of CMHC service requirements. The director of the resource coordination unit of the FSSA had documented many instances of unsuccessful referrals to the CMHC.

The FSSA administrator made this information available to the county human service planning agency after unsuccessful efforts to resolve the problem with the director of the mental health center. The CMHC, because of its high professional status and connections with the political power structure via its board members, did not feel obligated to work cooperatively with the lower-status and less-influential FSSA.

The community planning agency, under pressure from the administrator of the social service agency, decided to conduct a needs assessment of the services required by these severely disabled service consumers. The study concluded that the severely mentally disabled needed training in the skills of daily living, rather than the more traditional psychological counselling. It also determined that there was a potential training resource in the programs for the developmentally disabled and the severely physically handicapped.

The community planner, after learning of the referral problem arranged a meeting between the directors of the FSSA and the CMHC to discuss the reasons for the interagency conflict, and to determine whether there was a basis for cooperation. An examination of the goals of these two agencies showed that their official goals were compatible (i.e., the funding authorities of these two agencies required that they serve the severely disabled). However, there was disagreement on the operational level. The staff of the CMHC believed that the FSSA's service consumers were not appropriate for their agency's services.

In contrast with the lack of success in referring Betty Jones to the mental health center, the caseworker at the FSSA was more effective in linking her with a partial-care program that provided vocational training. The groundwork for this referral was laid by the resource coordination unit of the FSSA. The resource coordination unit was responsible for developing affiliation agreements with other agencies and supervising a community resource data bank that provided information on services available in the community. This unit had developed an agreement with the partial-care program that provided for a routine case conference on service consumers who were discharged from the county mental hospital. The staff of the partial-care program viewed the severely disabled as appropriate service users for their program.

Betty Jones' need for sheltered housing was not met because of the absence of this type of program in the community, although the State Department of Housing was exploring the possibility of legislation to remedy this problem. Various housing alternatives were being considered, including boarding homes and supervised apartments.

Mary was able to obtain financial assistance from the county welfare department. This successful referral was accomplished through the case coordinator's personal contacts with a staff member at the welfare department.

ISSUES

There are three issues relevant to community resource case coordination. One relates to the neglect of this interorganizational case-coordination function in direct service practice in general, and more specifically in the practice of case management. A second issue is associated with the relevance of this kind of intervention for service for severely disabled service consumer groups. The last issue concerns the professional risks associated with the advocacy role.

Community Resource Coordination and Direct-Service Practice

Case coordination is increasingly being recognized as an essential part of service to persons with a multiplicity of problems requiring resources from several agencies. It is a vital activity in case management (Moxley 1989:10). Welfare reform legislation in the Family Support Act of 1988 requires the coordination of such services as individual needs assessments and employability plans, job search, job development, placement services education, training, and support services, necessitating that the direct service person acquires specialized skills (Hagen and Wang 1993). A ten-state study of JOBS, the employment component of the Family Support Act, indicated that initial emphasis was placed on the broker or linkage function of case management (Hagen 1994).

Although the resource linkage function in direct practice has received some attention in recent years (Middleman and Goldberg 1974:65-72; Weisman 1987:47; Pincus and Minahan 1973:18-26; Rothman 1994), it has been underemphasized, particularly in case-management practice. Although the case-management literature has recognized the importance of resource linkage, various studies of case-management practice reveal that activities of case managers focus primarily on the service user and do not include tasks of interorganizational coordination (Austin, C. D. 1983:21; Austin, D. et al. 1980:38; Johnson and Rubin 1983:52-53). Rothman (1994) suggests that the referral function of direct practice is often a "marginal consideration in defining professional competency" (134). The need for more effective case coordination is indicated by evidence showing that only a small proportion of service consumers find the resources they seek when they are referred for service to other agencies (Cohen et al. 1980:3; Cummings 1968; Weisman 1976:52; Kirk and Greenley 1974:443). Studies of hospital discharge planning, which requires linkages to community resources, indicate that lack of connections with formal resources puts long-term patients at a greater postdischarge risk (Simon et al. 1995). Referral difficulties to the CMHC were evident in the case cited above.

One can speculate as to why direct practice has not given more recognition to the importance of resource linkage for the solution of problems facing their service users. There are at least two reasons: (1) an ideological bias that favors interventions directed at changing people rather than their environments (Neugeboren 1991:5-17); and (2) professional status that diminishes the importance of resource linkage as an essential part of professional practice (Johnson and Rubin 1983:50). A dominant philosophical inclination in direct practice favors interventions aimed at modifying service consumer attitudes and behavior. Textbooks in social work that claim a "generic" approach emphasize individual-change technologies (Schwartz 1977). Programs in social work education also focus on the individual (Thomas, C. H. 1983).

This ideological bias has been reinforced by the quest for professional status. Professional status in the helping professions has been identified with the fields of psychiatry and psychology. The quest for professional status has therefore led to the adoption of people changing technologies as the primary thrust of intervention. Consequently, the search for concrete resources and the process of referring service users to other agencies is an activity that has been relegated to less-trained staff on the assumption that this task requires less professional expertise (Johnson and Rubin 1983:50). It has not been appreciated that changing situations, including influencing policies and structures, requires knowledge and skill at least as complex as that needed for changing people (Johnson and Rubin 1983:53). Wolk, Sullivan, and Hartmann (1994) suggest that there are ten managerial roles performed in case management.

Relevance of Community Resource Coordination for the Severely Disabled

The emphasis in direct practice on changing individuals results from a failure to recognize that increasingly the kinds of persons requiring services suffer from severe disabilities that are not readily changed. Such social problems as child abuse, addiction, mental illness, mental retardation, crime, poverty, and illness associated with old age cannot be "cured" through individual-change interventions (Wintersteen 1986). Environmental modifications are usually more appropriate (Jansson 1984:427). Therefore, community resource coordination is especially relevant for service to the severely disabled who require a multiplicity of services from different specialized sources (Aiken et al. 1975:5; Kanter 1985; Rothman 1994). As illustrated in the case of Betty Jones, a severely mentally ill service user may need help finding employment, housing, medical care, and training in skills for independent living, which will necessitate the coordination of these services from different agencies.

Professional Risks of Client Advocacy in Resource Coordination

Consumer advocacy is frequently associated with case management (Fischer 1978; Lanoil 1980). The importance given to advocacy in social work is evident from the fact that the National Association of Social Workers' (NASW) endorsement of advocacy was derived from the NASW Code of Ethics (Ad Hoc Committee on Advocacy 1969). However, studies of professional practicee of advocacy indicate that it is limited (Jarrett and Fairbanks 1987). Internal agency advocacy was found to be somewhat common (Patti 1980; Rothman 1994), but external advocacy often exacted a personal price (burnout) from workers (Epstein 1981). Although professional integrity influences one to vigorously take sides (Rothman 1994:200), the practitioner also has to be aware of the possible negative consequences to his/her career.

Successful advocacy is associated with the use of communication and mediation rather than power (McGowan 1974). Advocacy operates best when relatively moderate means are used in situations involving modest conflict (Rothman 1994:202). A spectrum of adversarial tactics, varying with the intensity of conflict, has been identified, ranging from discussion, persuasion, and prodding to coercion (Rothman 1994:206). Organizational constraints on the advocacy role place the professional in a situation of conflicting interests: service user vs. professional vs. agency (Wolowitz 1983). The professional can be placed in a role conflict situation when s/he risks sanctions by confronting the agency's power structure. Power is most often the determining factor; the professional who lacks power to back up a confrontational advocacy stance risks organizational sanctions and, in extreme situations (e.g., whistleblowing), may be committing professional suicide (Westman 1991). The use of conflict tactics in the advocacy role is particularly problematic for human services students, because they have little authority to carry out this function. It is somewhat disingenuous for faculty to place the expectation of advocacy on students and future practitioners when they themselves will not risk performing this role.

Since power and authority are the keys to influencing others on behalf of the service user, the professional has to be skilled in developing and using power and authority (Kirst-Ashman and Hull 1993: 476-477; Neugeboren 1991:123-140).

The importance of power and authority in the process of obtaining resources for consumers of services has received little attention (Austin 1983). It would seem self-evident that the task of influencing autonomous agents to provide the needed services requires a level of legitimacy that is beyond that available to direct service staff. However, this authority can be provided through administrative structural supports (Rothman 1994:138-139). (See Chapter 5.)

The model of community resource coordination presented below assumes the use of a relatively low level of confrontation and conflict by use of such tactics as discussion and persuasion. It engages in such activities as: provider contracts; making needs known; use of nonaccusatory firmness; coaching service users; accompanying service consumers; accompanying service users and using knowledge of agency's policies and procedures (Rothman 1994:212).

DEFINITION OF COMMUNITY RESOURCE COORDINATION

Community resource coordination is an area of environmental practice that involves intervention in the interorganizational arena of the human services. In case management, it involves case coordination between agencies to accomplish service linkage for service consumers who require resources from several organizations. Community resource coordination is connected to environmental practice by its interorganizational context. Case coordination "occurs in a complex context–a broader reality comprising a multiplicity of organizations" (Austin 1981:4). Moxley (1989:22) describes this in terms of the indirect service function in case management, the objective of which is to change the system on behalf of the service user. Specifically, community resource coordination focuses on the *environmental barriers* that constrain the service user from receiving needed resources. For example, in the case cited above, the service consumer needed services from a social service agency, and a mental health center, a housing and financial assistance agency and a vocational rehabilitation agency. There were various barriers that hindered the service user from obtaining the required services, such as the absence of housing services and the reluctance of the CMHC to serve the severely disabled. In this situation, the task of the resource coordinator is to first understand the basis of these environmental barriers and then to develop strategies for overcoming them.

Resource Coordination as Systems Management

Resource coordination is conceived as "systems management," involving multilevel systems coordination (Levine and Fleming 1985:37; Sanborn 1983:8), and therefore requiring a "system's perspective" (Moxley 1989:143). A contradictory view is that community service delivery programs are "non-systems" (Netting 1992:160) lacking coherence and bouncing service users from agency to agency like a ping pong ball (U.S. General Accounting Office 1978).

The assumption of the model presented here is that, given the complexity of service systems, it is the obligation of human service practitioners to maximize the potentials for meeting service consumer needs. Moore (1992) sees service-delivery systems as having some rationality based on varying levels of service integration and resources. When service integration is high and resources are low, case management becomes a mechanism for rationing services. When both resources and integration are high, case management serves a marketing function. If resources are high and integration is low, case managers play a brokering role. If resources and integration are low, case management serves a developmental purpose.

This model is presented in terms of the potential for achieving an integrated service-delivery system.

The concept of systems management implies that responsibility and authority are vested in a single agency that will be held accountable for this service (Sanborn 1983:9). As indicated earlier, the different levels of resource coordination will be discussed in this chapter and the next. In line with the framework used here, Baumheier (1982:30-32) in a review of the literature identifies three major functions related to interagency coordination activities: (1) administration; (2) policy management and planning; and (3) direct service.

The role of administration is intertwined with case coordination because it provides the structural support that facilitates the interorganizational role of the resource case coordinator. Since case coordination is generally practiced under the auspices of direct service agencies, it requires administrative support to accomplish its tasks. This was illustrated in the case described above when the administrator of the resource coordination unit developed an affiliation agreement with the partial-care program that facilitated successful referral of the service consumer.

The relevance of community planning to resource coordination is related to the responsibility of planning and allocating agencies for facilitating service delivery coordination between the agencies they fund. This is evident in the case where the planning agency engaged in a needs assessment study to determine the availability of services for the severely mentally disabled.

An aspect of social policy formulation is designing policies that produce more effective and efficient service coordination. When gaps in service are present, it is the responsibility of the policy analyst to assist in formulating legislative policies that will make funding allocations contingent on the achievement of complementary service programs to fill the need. This role was elected in the case when the staff at the Department of Housing were in the process of developing policies to remedy the lack of housing services for the severely mentally ill.

The direct service role in community resource coordination will be the primary emphasis in this chapter. However, there is also a role for the community organizer, who, as an advocate for service users, is in a position to provide information to administrators, planners, and policy analysts on problems in service coordination. The community organizer, through contact with groups of community residents, is in an excellent position to learn of gaps in service coordination.

In summary, community resource coordination involves the actions of five kinds of professional staff: (1) the direct-service worker in case coordination; (2) the direct-service agency administrator, who provides the intraorganizational support for case coordination; (3) the community organizer, who receives information from groups of service consumers on service coordination deficiencies; (4) the community planner, who facilitates interagency coordination; and (5) the social policy analyst, who promotes policy formulation to aid in service coordination.

Community resource coordination involves three components: the community, resources, and the coordination process.

The Community

In community resource coordination, the community is the basic context for practice (Fellin 1987; Thomas and Shaftoe 1974; Froland et al. 1981:137-150). This community context includes the formal organizations and informal support systems that provide for basic needs of its residents. These resource systems range from the rate of vacant housing units to emergency health care facilities to neighborhood-based informal supports. In the assessment of the system of community care, attention is therefore focused on the network of these community services. The community "will be broadly conceived not as an obstacle to clients, but as a large pool of resources" (Rapp and Chamberlain 1985:419).

Intrinsic to this community-based practice is the knowledge of community structure and processes (Warren 1963). The structure of the community includes its heterogeneity, cultural traditions, population stability, and integrating institutions that influence its informal helping network (Froland et al. 1981:140-149). (See Chapter 5.) Knowledge of the community also implies an understanding of the location of the source of control of resources (Perlman and Gurin 1972:267), as well as the interorganizational structure that provides the basis for agency linkage (Lauffer 1978:187-238). With the community as the target for intervention, the resource coordinator has to understand and influence it in order to achieve more effective service for consumers.

In the Mary Smith case, the direct-service worker had to have an understanding of which community agencies provided the housing, vocational, and other kinds of services needed by the user. In addition, when confronted with the failure of referrals to the CMHC, the resource coordinator, the worker, the administrator, the planner, and the policy analyst had to understand how the power position of the its center influenced problems with the FSSA.

Resources

In contrast to the community agency resource *system* discussed above, we now highlight the specific resources exchanged in community resource coordination, such as, services, people, material, and strategic supports. Service resources include the available programs. People resources are the service consumers and staff in the agencies. Material includes money and other supports, such as facilities, equipment, and supplies. Strategic resources include such intangibles as power, status, legitimation, and professional expertise (Lauffer 1982:17).

As indicated, the community and its resources are assumed to provide an opportunity for the resource coordinator to link service users with needed resources. Despite the widespread belief that community resources are lacking, there is evidence of untapped resources and programs (Neugeboren 1979:180; Weisman 1976:51). Underutilization of community resources (Perlmutter, Heinemann, and Yudin 1974:31) occurs as a result of the complexity of community service systems and a lack of channeling mechanisms to access these service resources (Kahn 1969:162). In the case situation, services were available from the partial-care and financial-assistance programs. However, programs to teach the severely mentally ill the skills of daily living were underutilized.

Coordination

Coordination of services requires a the cooperative working relationship between agencies. A basic principle underlying interagency cooperation is *interorganizational dependency,* i.e, coordination is possible because the human-service agencies need each others resources to adequately serve consumers (Lauffer 1982). Two preconditions for agency interdependency are: (1) shared goals, and (2) resource interdependence (Reid 1965). Organizations will develop cooperative working relationships if their goals are congruent, rather than in conflict (Moxley 1989:101). They also need to be aware of the benefits to be derived from an exchange of resources. These benefits are the basis for influencing an organization to relinquish the autonomy required for successful coordination. In the case situation, the FSSA and the CMHC did not share operational goals and therefore did not perceive a need for each other's resources.

Community resource coordination occurs in three ways: (1) ad-hoc case coordination; (2) systematic case coordination; and (3) program coordination (Reid 1965:358). The type of coordination varies according to the extent of resource exchang and the impact on daily operations, including staff and agency autonomy.

Ad-hoc case coordination is the traditional means by which individual practitioners from different agencies refer service users to each other and exchange information when their cases overlap (Mathieson 1971). This type of coordination depends on the direct-service staff member's interest in coordination, as well as on the personal contacts he or she has with other workers. Since this is an individually determined activity, staff members tend to keep their information on community resources to themselves for use with their own service consumers. In the case, a personal contact was used to facilitate a referral to the financial assistance agency.

Systematic case coordination involves a more formalized process of coordinating services on a case basis, such as when two or more agencies agree on specific rules and a division of labor regarding referral procedures, information exchange, and routine case conferences. Systematic case coordination requires action on the part of administration to develop interagency agreements. This type of coordination is illustrated in the case in the relationship developed between the FSSA and the partial-care program.

Program coordination provides for the integration of two or more programs. Program coordination requires agreements on the policy level. Since it involves major modifications in staff activities, it is the most difficult type of coordination to accomplish. In the case, a joint program was developed between the FSSA and the county mental hospital whereby all patients discharged into the community received case-coordination services from the family agency.

INTERVENTIONS

Community Case Coordination

Up to this point, community resource coordination has been discussed in general terms with regard to issues and definitions. The focus will now shift to practice interventions on the micro, or case, level. Community resource case coordination is similar to "community service coordination" (Cohen et al. 1980) and linkage technology (Weisman 1976). Drawing on Cohen et al. (1980), community resource coordination involves three stages: (1) locating and selecting the appropriate community resource; (2) providing access and arranging for utilization of the preferred resource; and (3) supporting the service consumer's utilization of the resource and monitoring the outcome of the linkage efforts on service consumer's benefit. Community resource case coordination "expands the clients community support system by successfully linking the clients to an array of resources" (Cohen et al. 1980:1-2).

The linkage process requires the coordinator to identify and overcome the environmental barriers that interfere with effective referrals. Intrinsic to successful case coordination is the practitioner's responsibility to follow through until help for the service consumer is achieved (Cohen et al. 1980:7). This goal of case coordination precludes simple referrals that relieve the case coordinator of responsibility for the outcome (Weisman 1976:51). For the severely mentally ill, who cannot be "cured," the responsibility of the case coordinator is ongoing (Stein and Test 1980:392). Sanborn (1983:8-9) characterizes this as "total case management," where there is no "buck-passing," and where the case manager does not relinquish responsibility.

These three stages of community service coordination have been linked with specific activities. The following discussion describes the different activities associated with each of the stages of community service coordination, with emphasis on the environmental factors involved in this process. The skills needed to perform these activities will also be discussed.

These three major coordination activities are sequential and require specific steps to achieve the goals of each activity area. This model of case coordination separates the decision-making process of locating and selecting the appropriate resource from the plan for implementing this decision. It places considerable emphasis on the first stage (resource selection), since this is seen as a necessary precondition for the next two stages of decision implementation.

Stage I: Selecting the Appropriate Resource

Selecting the appropriate community resource requires the following sequence of activities by the case coordinator: (1) identifying service consumers' preferences and values; (2) identifying service users' community resource needs; (3) identifying the available community resources; (4) identifying viable community resource alternatives; (5) researching the potential community resource alternatives; and (6) choosing the appropriate community resource (Cohen et al. 1980:9-70).

Selecting the appropriate resource for the service consumer requires that the resource coordinator use *decision-making* skills, since this activity is related to the different aspects of problem solving. The activities of the three decision-making stages are conducted with different parties. Thus, problem definition is done primarily with the service user; the search for resource solutions is carried out with the resource unit; and cost/benefit evaluation is preformed with the aid of the supervisor.

Identifying the service consumer's needs and preferences involves the problem-definition stage of the decision-making process. Determination of resource alternatives relates to a search for potential solutions. Finally, researching and choosing the appropriate resource requires an evaluation of the relative costs and benefits of the various alternatives. The following chart illustrates the correspondence of the stages of decision making to the different activities involved in selecting the appropriate community resource, and with whom the activity is generally conducted.

SELECTING THE APPROPRIATE RESOURCE

STAGES OF DECISION MAKING	WITH WHOM CONDUCTED	ACTIVITIES INVOLVED
		Identifying of service user's preferences and values
Problem Definition	Service user	Identifying service user's community resource needs
		Identifying the available community resources
Search for Alternative Solutions	Resource unit	Identifying the viable resource alternatives
		Researching the potential resource alternatives
Evaluation of Cost/Benefit of Alternative Solutions	Supervisor	Choosing the appropriate resource

To *define the problem* confronted by the service consumer, the case coordinator needs to first *identify the service user's preferences,* which requires considerable involvement of the service consumer (Moxley 1989:98; Rothman 1994:143-145). In this process, one must be aware of the differences between service user "wants" and the professional perception of what they "need" (Goudenough 1963:49-60). The case coordinator will be under considerable pressure from service providers to influence the service consumer to do what they think is best in terms of his/her *needs* and, of special importance, in terms of *what the agency has to offer* (Rose

1992:272). The coordinator is in a position to force service users to go along with plans with which they may not agree. Given the lack of firm knowledge of *one* best path for service consumers to take, and since the user's motivation is a critical element, the coordinator can perform an important function of representing the service user's preferences by negotiating an agreement with other service providers that integrates both the wants and the needs of service consumers. This activity requires the case coordinator to utilize *representing* skills. In this instance, the service user's preferences need to be "marketed" to the provider by showing how the goals of the providers and the service consumer can be integrated. An *understanding of the service user's values and preferences* and representation of these interests to the provider can help avoid failure in resource linkage. The failure to achieve such an understanding was illustrated in the case, as the CMHC professionals referred the service consumer for psychological services, while the service user wanted concrete resources. Here, the case coordinator might have represented the service consumer's interests by influencing the professional to view the provision of concrete services as a first step in motivating the user to engage in a service program at the CMHC.

The situation in the case points to the general phenomenon that professionals tend to define service-user problems in terms of psychological needs in contrast to service consumers' desire for concrete resources (Goldberg and Warburton 1979:124; Neugeboren 1991:285-286; Pelton 1982; Webb and Wistow 1987:85). The CMHC staff emphasized Mary's motivational and psychological problems, while she perceive her primary problem to be the lack of a job. Therefore, in the case situation the resource case coordinator in utilizing the skill of decision making will first have to define the service consumer's problem in terms of whether it stems primarily from sources internal or external to the service user. Our concern with *environmental* barriers to effective service requires the case practitioner to use methods to overcome *external* impediments to the solution of service consumers' problems. Such external factors as "cost, availability, accessibility, and acceptability" can become barriers to service if they conflict with service users' preferences (Cohen et al., 1980:31). Rothman (1994:95-96) identifies key agency characteristics that may represent barriers to service utilization: the function of the agency; access and eligibility; fees; availability; quality and reliability; climate and accommodations; and key people in the system. Discussing the service consumer's wants and aspirations in relation to cost, availability, accessibility, and acceptability involves explaining what an exploration of preferences is, why it is important, and what is expected of the service user. In this process of eliciting the service consumer's preferences, it is essential that he or she understand the importance of being open in expressing preferences, so that the relevance of the service can be appreciated. Service users in general may be reluctant to express preferences openly for fear that their dissatisfactions may provoke such sanctions as being refused services.

The case coordinator needs to elicit the service consumer's preferences regarding cost, availability, accessibility, and acceptability so that these environmental barriers can be dealt with such that they are made congruent with service user's preferences. Related to these four preference areas are such issues as whether the service is beyond the economic means of the service consumer; the presence of waiting lists or lack of evening hours, which limit availability; physical accessibility in terms of transportation or accessibility in terms of language barriers; and acceptability in terms of the content of the program, its reputation, and its sensitivity to minorities. In the case, the service user did not keep appointments at the CMHC. The problem may have been that the service consumer found the service unacceptable, since she wanted help finding a job while the CMHC service stressed psychological treatment.

The next step in the problem-definition procedure requires the *identification of the resources needed by the service user.* This activity also should take into account environmental barriers to service. Failure of the service consumer to utilize a resource typically is attributed to his/her disability or deficiencies. In contrast, environmentally oriented case coordination would explore the *failure of the resource* to meet the service user's needs. Resource failure can be attributed to the "inappropriateness of the service or the unacceptability of the manner, method, or context in which it is delivered" (Cohen et al. 1980:10). In the case, the worker's definition of the problem would have determined that the psychotherapeutically oriented environment of the CMHC was inappropriate for the service needs of this severely disabled service consumer.

The determination of the kinds of resources required by the service user involves a resource assessment. "A resource assessment is an evaluation of the supports needed for a client to achieve the overall rehabilitation goal. An understanding of available supports clarifies the resources the client can rely on to succeed in the specified environment" (Anthony, Nemec, and Cohen 1987). Types of resources assessed include people, places, things, and activities. Moxley (1989:54) compiled a resource matrix form that synthesizes assessment information on twelve need areas with evaluations of self-care, mutual care and professional care capacities. In the case, a resource assessment would determine the kind of environmental supports the service user needed to succeed in the programs in which she was engaged. These might include transportation to assure that the service consumer could attend the training classes and financial assistance from the welfare department to meet economic needs.

The next step involves the *identification of available community resources*, including the ones that are *viable alternatives* (i.e., those that will meet the service user's need and for which the service consumer is eligible). This step relates to the search-for-alternative-solutions stage of the decision-making process. Identification of community resources involves obtaining listings of and essential information on formal agency services, as well as information about informal support network resources. One approach to obtaining resource listings involves securing information from funding authorities, such as the United Way, who may have centralized information and referral programs. The community resource case coordinator needs to have knowledge of such essential information as the particular mandate or mission of each community resource with which she or he is working (Cohen et al. 1980:7). In the case, it was important for the case coordinator to be aware that the mandate of the partial-care program was congruent with the service needs of the service user because of its goal serving the severely disabled mentally ill.

Rapid and efficient access to information on community resources requires the case coordinator to have a system for storing and retrieving this information. One way of organizing resource information is to create folder or card files according to resource areas (e.g., housing, medical care, etc.). Since the task of collecting and updating comprehensive information on community resources may be too much to expect of individual case coordinators, the agency should provide this through a data bank (Rothman 1994:91) in a resource coordination unit as was done in the Mary Smith case. (See Chapter 5 for a discussion of the functions of the resource coordination unit.)

Identification of viable community resources alternatives requires obtaining "inside" information that is not readily available from public sources. Information can be obtained from written or personal sources. Written sources include the case coordinator's resource file, enriched by information from service providers. Personal sources include colleagues, supervisors, and other service consumers. Information obtained from colleagues, supervisors, and service users will usually include program evaluation data that is not available from written sources. An example of this is information on the distinction between the "official" and "operative" goals and structures of agencies (Neugeboren 1991:30). To facilitate service consumer entry into community service programs, the case coordinator needs to know how the "operative" intake policies *fit* the "official" policies and procedures described in resource directories. Another type of useful "unofficial" information is the circumstances under which the agency will bend eligibility requirements.

Since the information required to identify viable community resources can be contained through an agency's resource coordination unit, the case coordinator will generally work with the staffperson from this unit to identify available resources. In the case, there was a discrepancy between the "official" and "operative" goals of the CMHC. The case coordinator might have communicated this discrepancy to the resource coordinator supervisor, who could have taken this up with his counterpart at the CMHC.

The process for establishing service user eligiblility for the available services involves the matching of the service requirements with service consumer characteristics. Service requirements usually are defined in terms of such service user characteristics as age, sex, income level, and geographical residence. Here again, service eligibility can be assessed not only in terms of the official requirements in terms of the conditions under which exceptions to these written requirements are made. Case coordinators can obtain exceptions for their service consumers after developing working relationships with colleagues in other agencies. The resource coordination unit may also have information as to the kinds of rule deviations possible in the different agencies.

Researching the community resource alternatives and choosing the appropriate one is the last step of Stage I of community case coordination. It corresponds to the last stage of the decision-making process, evaluation of the cost/benefit of alternative solutions. This activity will often require assistance from a supervisor in arriving a final decision as to the most appropriate resource for the service user.

Researching community resource alternatives involves the determination of the extent to which these resources are able to satisfy the service consumer's preferences. A comparative evaluation is conducted of the compatibility of each resource with the service user's interests, with the final decision determined by which resource is most congruent with his/her preferences (Weisman 1976:52). For example, evaluating the relative costs of alternative programs provides information that can be used to decide which programs are compatible with service consumer's preference on expense.

Choosing the appropriate resource depends upon a determination of which alternative will best meet the service consumer's needs and wants. Since this decision-making process depends upon an understanding of the service user's values and preferences, service consumer involvement is essential to facilitate this process.

In situations where the resource selected is not congruent with the service user's preferences, a recycling of the decision is required. In that instance, there are three possible ways to develop a viable alternative: (1) modifying an existing resource; (2) reconsidering alternative resources; and (3) developing new resources.

Modifying an existing resource involves working with a resource and/or service consumer to overcome the resource's deficits. In the case, the deficits of the CMHC could have been overcome by the case coordinator exerting influence on the CMHC to modify their approach to the service user by responding to Mary Smith's desire for concrete services. This might be accomplished by convincing them to give first priority to service user's vocational and housing goals by arranging for training in word processing and expediting a placement in a living situation which she could afford.

Reconsidering alternative resources means determining whether there are other resources that may be more congruent with the service consumer's preferences. In the case, the coordinator could have explored the availability of another CMHC that had a program that provided concrete services.

Developing new resources goes beyond the scope of the authority of the case coordinator. Nevertheless, it is possible for a case coordinator to contribute to resource developement within the community by feedback through the supervisor to relevant community groups (e.g., institutions that fund resources, advocacy groups) responsible for ensuring that adequate resources exist. In the case, the coordinator gave information to the supervisor on the inadequacy of the CMHC program for the severely disabled, which was subsequently passed on to the community planning agency.

Stage II: Arranging for Service User Utilization of the Preferred Resource

Arranging for the service consumer's utilization of the preferred resource involves connecting to the resource, which includes the activities of "(1) preparing to make the resource aware of the client's need; (2) obtaining the agreement of the resource to provide the service; (3) finalizing the arrangements to utilize the resource to provide service; (4) developing a program to utilize the resource" (Cohen et al. 1980:71-98). These linkage activities depend heavily on the ability of the case coordinator to negotiate agreements with the resource provider. Therefore, *negotiating* skills will be needed, meaning that the case coordinator will have to find complementary interests between the parties derived from shared goals and resource exchange. In the case, successful referral to the partial-care program was facilitated because the two agencies shared similar goals.

However, the ability to negotiate successfully will also be affected by the legitimacy and authority of the case coordinator (Morris 1977:357; Neugeboren 1991:284-285), which in turn is dependent on the structural supports provided by the agency policies and procedures. Rothman (1994:138-139) cites different types of authority, including administrative, legal, and fiscal, that are needed to facilitate the linkage of service users to formal organizations. In the case, the successful referral to the partial-care program was facilitated by the structural support provided by interagency agreement between the FSSA and that program. (Administrative supports for case coordination are discussed in Chapter 5.)

The process of *preparing to make the resource aware of the service user's need* (Moxley 1989:99) will be enhanced if the case coordinator formulates specific and operational statements on the expectations of outcomes. This is accomplished when outcomes are defined in terms of specific resources and skills needed by the service user, rather than in terms of diagnostic labels, symptoms, or attitudes. In the case, a successful outcome would be the service consumer obtaining appropriate housing and vocational skills. The formulation of outcomes should lead to the specification of program characteristics that can achieve these desired outcomes. This is illustrated in the case where Mary Smith expressed interest in developing a skill in word processing. The case coordinator should refer her to a program that taught this skill.

The next step, *obtaining the agreement of the resource to provide service*, requires the linking of a need and resource self-interest. Some benefits to a resource may be: (1) obtaining new funds; (2) receiving positive publicity and good will (Moxley 1989:102); (3) accomplishing an agency mandate; and (4) increasing productivity and efficiency. This step involves use of the *negotiating* skill, the success of which is dependent on the potential for the exchange of resources. Influencing the resource to provide the service therefore depends on an interdependency derived from shared goals (Zald 1965) and resource exchange. This occurred in the case situation, where the partial-care program, which was mandated to serve the severely disabled mentally ill, needed referrals of this type of service consumer.

Another way of appealing to the self-interest of the resource is for the case coordinator to identify the service user's assets relative to the program's goals. These assets need to be presented in a way that assures that the referral goal can be accomplished. In the case, the high motivation of the service consumer for vocational training should be emphasized.

Anticipating and responding to a resource's objections and concerns about the referral of a service user is another way of reconciling consumer need and resource self-interest. The coordinator will want to prepare responses to the objections of the resource in advance. In the case of the mentally ill, these objections may stem from deficits (e.g., repeated hospitalizations) or from the resource's own situation (e.g., staff anxiety regarding potential danger of discharged mental patients). In the former instance, the coordinator can point to lack of previous effort to prepare the service user for community adjustment. The latter objection can be dealt with by providing information that discharged mental patients are no more dangerous than other groups in the community. The general perception that mental patients are dangerous results from the prominence given to mental health status by the news media when mental patients commit serious crimes (Mechanic 1980:200).

The linking of consumer need and resource self-interest also involves *representing skills*. The case coordinator must address the service consumer's needs in relationship to the resource service eligibility requirements. For example, if the policy of the CMHC requires that the service consumer first have individual counseling sessions in order to be eligible for concrete services, then this has to be told to the service user. The coordinator must "sell" the agency services to the user in terms that are relevant to his/her needs. The direct service supportive role is enhanced by the case coordinator's representing skills, which capitalize on the mutual interests of the service consumer and the community resource.

Finalizing the arrangements to utilize the resource involves negotiating an agreement that specifies the desired results, the services expected to achieve that outcome, and the part to be played by the case coordinator. This agreement can be formalized at a *linkage meeting* attended by the service user, the coordinator, and an agency representative (Moxley 1989:99). A written agreement or contract provides a framework that can facilitate the implementation of the roles and responsibilities of the different parties involved (Moxley 1989:102). In the case, an agreement could be formulated with regard to Mary Smith's goal of learning word processing skills, with the case coordinator agreeing to provide transportation to the classes and the partial-care program providing the required educational programming.

The affiliation agreement between the FSSA and the partial-care program provided the basis for a contract to provide the specific services needed by the user, including the expected outcomes of vocational skills and job placement. Again, the successful accomplishment of this outcome relies on the case coordinator being aware of the self-interests of the other party to insure that these interests are met in the negotiation process.

Developing a program to utilize the resource requires the anticipation of potential resource problems that could hinder the service consumer's successful utilization of the resource. Program personnel are a critical resource that should be assessed in terms of compatibility for needs. This is especially the case in programs for the severely disabled, since many staff in the human services have not been trained to work with this population. The resource case coordinator can assist in this situation by reminding the resource of the severe nature of the problems and the need to adjust expectations accordingly. Since it is unlikely that staff who are not trained to serve the severely disabled will learn new intervention skills, it is important that these service users be referred to agencies that can meet their needs. In the case, the coordinator should consult with the resource coordination unit to determine which agencies have the capability of working with this type of service user. In Mary Smith's case, it might have been better if she had not been referred to the CMHC, given the lack of fit between their services and her needs.

Stage III: Supporting Utilization of the Resource

The tools used in supporting the service user's utilization of the resource have been referred to as "cementing techniques" (Weissman 1976:53). This stage involves ensuring that those responsible carry through on the necessary steps to successfully implement the service consumer's utilization of the resource. Necessary actions include "(1) developing time lines for action; (2) developing reenforcers to ensure action; (3) monitoring performance; and (4) modifying the program to improve its effectiveness" (Cohen et al. 1980:99-108).

Developing Time Lines. Time lines specify when something is to be done and when it will be completed. It permits the coordinator and service user to monitor progress in resource utilization. Time lines asist in the early identification of problems. In the case, time lines could have been established for the referral of Mary to the CMHC, which would have resulted in an early identification of the problem of lack of fit between the expectations of the service consumer and the CMHC. In addition, the coordinator could develop specific time lines for referrals in accordance with the service user's objectives regarding living arrangements. Perhaps a time-limited placement in a boarding home could precede placement in a supervised apartment.

Developing Reinforcers to Ensure Action. Reinforcers are actions that motivate the service user to fulfill responsibilities. If the cause of the service-delivery problem is that the goals of the program are too distant, then reinforcers should be linked to the program steps to achieve the goals.

Monitoring. Monitoring is used to determine if utilization is occurring in accordance with the plan. The monitoring process involves six substeps: "(1) identifying what is to be monitored; (2) identifying who is to do the monitoring; (3) identifying where the monitoring is to be done; (4) identifying when the monitoring is to be done; (5) identifying how the monitoring is to be done; and (6) identifying how learning from the monitoring is to be shared" (Cohen et al. 1980:103). In the case situation, monitoring of the referral for housing would follow the above steps to ensure the success of the referral. Once the service user is referred, the case coordinator should closely monitor the kinds of services being provided in order to insure that expectations are appropriate (Moxley 1989:114-123; Rothman 1994:172-198).

Modifying the Program. The monitoring results will determine whether a modification of the program is needed. In the case situation, referral to the partial care program represented a modification of the initial program of referral to the CMHC.

Actions such as developing time lines, reinforcement actions, monitoring, and program modification must be done within the context of interorganizational agreements, which provide the authority for ensuring that proper implementation will occur. Especially where program modification is required, agency agreements will be used as a means for achieving change. If the policies governing interorganizational agreements are found to be deficient, then it is the case coordinator's responsibility to make this known to the administrator, who can take steps to rectify the problem. In the case situation, the lack of housing-placement resources made it necessary for the administrator of the FSSA to renegotiate with the partial-care program for the inclusion of these services.

Contextual Influences on Case Decision Making

The above model of community resource case coordination should be supplemented with an understanding of how the organizational environment influences case decision making. The power of the agency *context*–its goals, structure, philosophy, and technologies–to affect case decision making needs to be understood if the resource coordinator is to be effective (Neugeboren 1991:172). Lack of appreciation of contextual influences on case coordination can subvert the process. The impact of the agency environment will be illustrated in the resource allocation process that is intrinsic to any service-delivery procedure.

Resource Allocation

The contextual influences on case coordination are evident in decision making that occurs during the resource allocation process. Resource allocation by the case coordinator involves three phases: screening, assessment, and care planning (Austin 1981). This process occurs within the context of the agency's goals, structures, ideologies, and resources. In general, agencies will tend to be biased toward screening, assessing, and implementing service plans in terms of its goals, structures, ideologies, and technologies. This phenomenon is connected to the *nonrational* aspect of the decision-making process, i.e., agency context will constrain a *rational* effort to solve problems. This was illustrated in the case situation in the CMHC intake policies, which were influenced by a staff preference for service to less-disabled users, who they viewed as more "motivated." These operational goals subverted the official goals of service to the severely mentally ill.

Implementation of the three phases of resource allocation by the case coordinator requires the use of decision-making skills. The following discussion illustrates how these skills are linked to the activities and tasks of resource allocation (case screening, assessment, and planning) within the organizational context associated with this process.

Screening, which involves determining eligibility for services, is related to the agency's need to maintain and defend its domain. Agency domain (turf) refers to the area of responsibility claimed by the agency (i.e., the kinds of users it serves and the types of services it provides). The decision-making process for screening can easily impact on other agencies and result in conflict if there is not agreement between agencies as to who legitimately should be serving which users (domain consensus).

In the case situation, there was a problem in referring cases to the CMHC. In applying the *decision-making* skill, the case coordinator first has to *formulate the problem* in order to determine the cause of the difficulty. The coordinator might arrive at the following two alternative problem formulations: (1) lack of clarity in agency policies regarding each agency's respective roles and responsibilities in providing services to the severely disabled mentally ill, or (2) poor communication among the staff members involved in the particular case.

Assuming the problem was defined as lack of clarity in agency policies, two possible alternative solutions are: (1) developing a long-term solution through an interagency agreement; or (2) developing a short-term solution where by the staff engaged in the conflict would clarify their respective roles and responsibilities in the particular case situation in order to arrive at a case plan that they agree would be beneficial to the specific user.

The next step in decision making involves the *evaluation of the costs and benefits of alternative solutions* to the problem. The decision maker will determine which of the alternative solutions should be used based on which alternative achieved the most benefit at the least cost. In the example given, one could anticipate that, in terms of staff involvement, the costs associated with the second alternative (case solution) will be less than those of the first alternative (policy solution). However, benefit will be greater in the second alternative, since a policy change will affect a larger number of service users. If the case coordinator is interested in having an impact beyond the particular case, then he or she will probably opt for the second alternative. However, the case coordinator's lack of power limits his or her ability to influence policy directly. Here, the case coordinator is required to feed the information back to administrative personnel who are in a position to take the necessary steps to influence a change in policy.

Service user *assessment* involves gathering data to determine the service consumer's needs and wants. Here again, there is potential for viewing the service consumer's needs in terms of the kinds of services available in the particular agency. To insure that the service consumer's "wants" are being considered, it may be necessary to establish some mechanism for feedback. This is facilitated by involving in the assessment procedure a service user appeal process involving an independent party such as an ombudsman. If such a mechanism was available at the CMHC, then the subversion of the official goals of service to the severely mentally ill might have been avoided.

Care planning translates the assessment data into a service plan, which results in the allocation of resources for the user. It includes determining the service needs of the consumer, contacting service providers, arranging for services, and explaining the plan to the serivce user. Rothman (1994:103-110) proposes the following criteria for designing a strategy of implementation planning: feasibility, effectiveness, acceptability, and implementability. Plan implementation involves such principles as individualization of service; comprehensiveness of service; parsimony of service; fostering empowerment; and continuity of care.

Care planning is similar to the three stages of community service coordination discussed above (i.e., selecting, arranging for utilization, and supporting utilization of resources). Accordingly, there is the potential danger of limiting care plans to the services available within the agency, as well as a potential for bias in screening and assessment.

This problem of agency context producing distortions in the resource allocation process can be dealt with by the establishment of rules that rely on objective criteria for decision making in screening, assessment and care planning. Although professionals tend to resist efforts to standardize their practice, rules can be established based on practice experience, as has been done in hospital care utilization committees (Austin et al. 1980). For example, procedures that support preference would counteract the tendency of the agency context to subvert users' wants.

Another way of minimizing contextual bias is to place the responsibility for the three functions of screening, assessment, and care planning with separate persons or organizational units. However, the resource case coordinator should be aware that the organizational context can have a pervasive influence on the decision-making process.

It has been suggested that the resource case coordinator can potentially modify the service delivery system through feedback of information to administrators on problems in interorganizational relations, e.g., conflict over agency domain. Information on gaps in services can be made available to community planners via the administrative structure of the agency. Although some believe that ad-hoc resource coordination can have a cumulative effect on patterns of interdependence between agencies (Austin 1983:17), others indicate that it has little effect because the resource case coordinator lacks authority (Austin 1983:22-23).

Since resource case coordination is practiced within direct service agencies, administrators need to provide the structural support needed to facilitate this function. The roles of the administrator, the planner, and the policy analyst in resource coordination will be discussed in Chapter 5.

SUMMARY

This chapter reviewed the underlying issues of community resource coordination, and defined some of the relevant concepts. Resource coordination was viewed in systems terms, so that interventions on the micro and macro levels were deemed necessary.

A case example was used to illustrate the skills and interventions required in community resource case coordination. Three kinds of coordination activities included: (1) locating and selecting the appropriate community resource; (2) providing access to and arranging for utilization of the preferred resource; and (3) supporting utilization of the resource, including follow-up to monitor the benefit of the linkage efforts. The constraining effects of the organizational context on the resource allocation process of screening, assessment, and care planning was also discussed. Throughout, the focus has been on the *environmental* barriers that need to be overcome in successful practice of community resource coordination.

The next chapter discusses community resource coordination on the macro level and how it is linked to coordination on the case level.

STUDY QUESTIONS

1. You are the case coordinator working for the FSSA and have difficulty referring Mary Smith to the CMHC. What action would you take to resolve the problem?

2. In order to resolve the problem of referral to the CMHC, what specific skill(s) will be required?

3. As case coordinator of the FSSA, what would you do after you discovered the differences between the official and operative goals of the CMHC?

4. As case coordinator, you have become aware that the professional ideologies of your colleagues at the FSSA constrain the service you are trying to provide to the severely disabled mentally ill. What would you do about this?

5. Indicate some of the environmental barriers that had to be overcome in the case situation.

6. Indicate how administrative support facilitated the efforts of the case coordinator.

7. Using the case, discuss how the interdependence of the FSSA and partial-care program facilitated their joint efforts. Focus your discussion on the concepts of shared goals and resource exchange.

8. What resources, if any, might have been exchanged between the FSSA and the CMHC?

Chapter 5

COMMUNITY RESOURCE COORDINATION ON THE MACRO LEVEL

Community Resource Coordination on the Macro Level

INTRODUCTION

This chapter on community resource coordination on the macro level includes separate discussions of the roles of administrators of direct-service agencies, planners in community-planning organizations, and social policy analysts in policy-formulating agencies. As indicated previously, an understanding of macro practitioner roles and responsibilities is important not only for administrators, planners, and policy analysts, but also for case coordinators. Effective case coordination requires a full understanding by direct service staff of the macro functions that facilitate their performance on the case level. Thus, case coordinators should be aware of their role of providing feedback on such case-coordination problems as agency reluctance to accept legitimate referrals and gaps in service resources.

The various skills required by the macro practitioner will be illustrated in this chapter through application to the case situation described at the beginning of Chapter 4.

ISSUES

There are two problems that confront the macro practitioner in the successful achievement of community resource coordination. The first is the failure to recognize the interdependency between the macro and micro levels of community resource coordination. The second problem is the structural barriers that hinder the planner and policymaker from achieving interorganizational coordination in an effective manner.

Interdependency of Macro and Micro Community Resource Coordination

A basic issue in the practice area of community resource coordination relates to the lack of recognition of the interdependency between micro and macro levels. Practitioners on the case level need the support of administrators, planners, and policymakers in order to obtain the resources and authority needed to create linkages between autonomous agencies. "For the practitioner to move forward with specific clients, a platform has to be put in place involving system-level functions, largely carried forward by administrators and policy makers" (Rothman 1994:219). O'Connor (1988) also views case management as a multilevel system requiring micro and macro staff to perform different and related roles, functions, and technologies. This organizational support is critical to ensure service user access. Without such access, programs exist merely as monuments to good intentions lacking practical utility for the consumers (Moore 1990:447). Conversely, macro practitioners are dependent on the direct-service staff for information on the gaps, deficiencies, and barriers to effective service. Observation of actual micro and macro practice suggests that these two areas are conducted somewhat independently of each other.

In fact, it appears that there may be a certain amount of alienation (Lauffer 1978:33) and conflict between these two levels of practice, rooted in different values and practice philosophies (Patti and Austin 1977). The micro practitioner can often be heard complaining that administrators do not appreciate the constraints confronting the line workers in their attempts to coordinate services. Administrators, planners, and policymakers criticize the direct-service worker for not understanding the political barriers (e.g., turf protectiveness) that prevent better coordination.

This conflict between macro and micro levels of practice tends to hide a basic interdependency between these two practice levels based on (1) the micro practitioner's need for macro support to facilitate case coordination, and (2) the macro practitioner's need for feedback from the operational level to facilitate more effective administration, planning, and policymaking. The following material is intended to increase the awareness of both micro and macro level practitioners of their interdependency so there can be more cooperation between these two levels of practice.

Micro Practitioners' Need for Macro Support

As was indicated in the previous chapter, the practice of community resource case coordination has not recognized the need for administrative, planning, and policy support for the direct service practitioner. Although the social science literature has studied and analyzed issues in the interorganizational arena (Aiken et al. 1975; Litwak and Rothman 1970; Hasenfeld 1983: 59-82), this theory and research has not often been linked with direct practice. Exception is the work of Lauffer (1982:187-238) and Rothman (1994: 134-171), which specifies a variety of interagency linkages at the operational level.

One has to wonder at the lack of attention devoted to the role and responsibility of administrative, planning, and policy practitioners in community resource case coordination given the need for authority and power concomitant to the task of coordinating services among agencies (Rothman 1994:138-139). One explanation may be that human service organizations have been reluctant in general to engage in agency coordination and integration. Turf protectiveness, ideological differences, and funding sources that facilitate specialized rather than integrated programs have been some of the reasons for the lack of interagency coordination (Hasenfeld 1983:50; Lauffer 1982:187; Morris and Lescohier 1978:21-50; Neugeboren 1991:220-222). Upper-level authority has therefore left to the line practitioner with the responsibility for coordinating services on the case level. Consequently, this places the direct-service worker in the untenable position of having the responsibility for interagency case coordination without the necessary authority (Neugeboren 1991:284).

Macro Practitioners' Need for Micro Feedback

As indicated above, administrators, planners, and policymakers frequently function in isolation from the problems and issues that commonly arise on the direct-service level. The nature of organizational life precludes efficient communication of information between the line and upper levels (Hall 1977). Similarly, communication between the line practitioner and planning and policy practitioners is constrained by the lack of linkages between direct service and planning and policy organizations. The result is that official and operative policies are frequently incongruent (Neugeboren 1991:62-63).

This kind of communication problem was evident in the case situation. The director of the CMHC was surprised to learn at the meeting with the community planner that the CMHC staff, contrary to official policy, were restricting services to the severely mentally ill.

Structural Constraints on Community Planners' Efforts to Achieve Interagency Coordination

Traditionally, a role and function of community planning agencies has been to coordinate services (Perlman and Gurin 1972: 195; Lauffer 1982:75-76). The operating guidelines of planning organizations like the United Way mandate planning, allocating funds, and the coordination of the services they finance. However, their coordination role is constrained by their "federated" structures. Their boards consist of representatives of the provider agencies they fund (Rein and Morris 1962), which constrains their power and authority to coordinate the organizations on which they are dependent (Lauffer 1978:39; Perlman and Gurin 1972:198). Such structural constraints have implications for the kinds of practice skills that are needed on the macro level. Specifically, community planners need to use leadership, negotiating, and representing skills to accomplish the interagency collaboration that is necessary for successful community resource coordination. This will be illustrated below in a discussion of administration, planning, and policy roles in relation to the case.

INTERVENTIONS

Organizational Level: Administration of Direct-Service Agencies

As indicated in the model for administration of direct-service organizations (see Chapter 1), three major tasks need to be accomplished: formulation of organizational goals; design of agency structures; and implementation of programs. In the area of community resource coordination, the *formulation of organizational goals* with an environmental focus is a precondition for the subsequent tasks of program design and implementation.

As participants in the *design of agency structures,* administrators are responsible for developing administrative supports within their agencies that will facilitate interorganizational case coordination. (Aiken et al. 1975). Structures are required to facilitate the resource case coordinator's work in the interorganizational arena. Middleman and Goldberg (1974:69) argue for a universalistic perspective that goes beyond crisis-oriented case coordination and that develops structures that will endure beyond any single service user. These policies relate to intra- and interorganizational structures that provide the framework for interorganizational case coordination (Austin et al. 1980:51). These structural supports are required to ensure that the case coordinator has the authority and sanction needed to obtain the required resources for the service consumer (Austin 1983:17; Austin et al. 1980:54; Neugeboren 1991:284). This authority can be achieved through administrative, legal, and fiscal means (Rothman 1994: 138-139). Administrative authority and control is conferred on the practitioner by the definition of roles and responsibilities. Legal authority is achieved through legislative mandates. Fiscal authority is accomplished through the purchase of services on behalf of the service user. One type of administrative structure that can facilitate the case coordinator role is the resource coordination unit.

Resource Coordination Unit

The administrative task of *implementing programs* require the establishment of a resource coordination unit. This is an organizational unit whose function is to provide the support required by direct-service workers to coordinate services for individual cases (Aiken et al. 1975). This staff unit needs the specialized knowledge and skill to intervene in the interorganizational arena of practice. Specific skills include decision making, negotiating, monitoring, representing, and staffing. These skills are employed by the resource coordination unit to fulfill the following tasks: (1) determine the unmet service needs of the service consumers being served by the agency (decision making; monitoring); (2) locate agencies through the development of agency profiles (monitoring) that dispense services that are unavailable within the unit's organization and which are needed by their service users; (3) negotiate agreements to exchange resources (representing; negotiating); and (4) facilitate an interagency understanding of each other's programs through cross-agency training (staffing) (Neugeboren 1987:8-9).

Determining Unmet Service Needs. Program implementation requires ascertaining the unmet service needs of the service users. This necessitates an information system that routinely monitors caseloads to determine gaps in services. The administrative staff uses skills in monitoring, that including program-evaluation activities, to determine unmet service needs. This involves systematic follow-up on service outcomes to identify the causes of service deficiencies. Information on barriers to effective service outcomes can be obtained from line staff, as well as from service consumers. The resource coordination unit determines from this information the types of services are needed but not available, as well as any discrepancies between official and operative agency goals.

This process is illustrated in the case situation where the resource coordination unit used monitoring skills when they collected information on service gaps for the severely mentally ill. Decision-making skills were used in determining the reason for this service deficiency. The unit then discovered that the reluctance of the CMHC to serve this service user group was associated with the conflicting expectations of the service consumers and the clinical staff.

Locating Agencies that Can Fill Service Gaps. Program implementation also requires locating agencies that can fill these service gaps. This necessitates the ongoing collection and storage of information on the kinds of services available in the community (Lauffer 1982: 30-46; Rothman 1994:93; Weisman 1976:52), a process that requires monitoring skills. This counters the general practice of direct-service workers, who often develop a personal resource file that is not made available to other staff and their service users. The resource coordination unit's task is to actively seek out resources, some of which may be hidden (Perlmutter, Heinemann, and Yudin 1974:31), and to make sure that all workers and service consumers have equal access to information about these services.

Another reason for an agency to develop its own resource data system is that community data systems (e.g., resource directories) become outdated quickly, since programs are in constant flux (Rothman 1994:94). In addition, community resource directories provide information on *official* agency goals, but lack data on the *operative* goals. An agency resource data bank can provide both types of information. In order to successfully refer cases, staff should know not only what an agency's official policy is in regard to service user eligibility for their services, but also what the actual intake practice is in terms of the types of service consumers actually *preferred.* This distinction was illustrated in the case, where the CCMHC's official policy was to serve the severely mentally ill, while in actual practice it gave preference to less-disabled service users who were more "motivated" for service. (See the Appendix for sample agency profile outline.)

Information on agencies that can be useful in accessing resources are the function of agency; eligibility criteria; availability; quantity and reliability; climate (user friendliness); and the names of people in the system who control decisions about acceptance for service (Rothman 1994:95-96). Agency profiles should also show the kinds of service resources available within the organizational set of the particular agency. The organizational set refers to those specific agencies with which an organization shares or has the potential to share resources (Lauffer et al. 1977:47). The information in these agency profiles enables the resource coordination unit to determine potentials for resource exchange. This information provides the basis for the resource coordination unit's negotiation of interagency service agreements.

Negotiation of Interagency Agreements. The promotion of inter-agency agreements is an important program-coordination strategy (Netting et al. 1990; Neugeboren 1991:220). These formal agreements can help establish domain consensus (i.e., agreement between those that control access to resources) (Hasenfeld 1983:63). Lack of formal agreements between human service agencies can be a barrier to access to resources external to the agency (Austin et al. 1980:46-47). Two types of agreements have been utilized: affiliations and liaisonships (Neugeboren 1987:8). *Affiliation* agreements are broad policy statements created between agency directors that indicate an intent for the two agencies to cooperate. *Liaisonship* agreements are more specific agreements delineating the procedures for referral and conflict resolution between two agencies. The affiliation agreement, involving the higher administrative levels, facilitates the development of the more specific operational liaisonship agreements. (See the Appendix for sample affiliation and liaisonship agreements.)

Administrative linkages consist of fiscal agreements (joint budgeting, joint funding, and purchase of services); personnel practices (consolidated personnel administration, staff transfers, staff sharing, and co-location of staff); planning and programming (joint planning, programming, evaluation, and information exchange); and administrative support services (joint recordkeeping, grant management, and central support services) (Streeter et al. 1986).

The type of affiliation agreement used is affected by the coordination strategies, of which there are three types: mutual adjustment, alliance, and corporate (Mulford and Rogers 1982). Mutual adjustment strategies focus on specific cases, tend to be informal, and involve the fewest costs for the participating organization (Reid 1965). Alliance strategies involve formal or informal collaboration for the accomplishment of mutual organizational goals. Corporate strategies are more formalized, with the power vested in the upper levels of administration. This is similar to program coordination (Reid 1965).

Promulgation of interagency agreements requires the use of representing and negotiating skills. Representing skill is used by the resource coordination staff to communicate to the target agency the kind of information needed to understand the nature of the organization's program (such as its goals and type of users served). Representing activities are naturally linked with negotiating efforts, which are dependent on making visible the extent to which both agencies have shared goals and can benefit from a mutual exchange of resources.

The development of an interagency affiliation agreement is illustrated in the case situation by the resource unit's development of an agreement with the partial-care program. This agreement was facilitated by the fact that both agencies had shared goals (service to severely mentally ill service consumers) and could benefit from an exchange of staff resources at routine case conferences.

Cross-Agency Training. The *implementation* of interagency coordination can be enhanced by cross-agency training, which facilitates better understanding of each agency's services. Cross training involves two agencies agreeing to allow their staff to participate in the in-service training programs of the other agency (Lauffer 1982:55). This device allows staff to obtain firsthand knowledge of the policies and practice procedures operating in the other agency. Cross training is a mechanism for breaking down the barriers of interagency communication.

In-service training requires staffing skills. Staffing skills are dependent on the integration of individual and organizational goals (Neugeboren 1991:76-78). Agency personnel responsible for in-service training should be able to identify how the abilities, skills, and interests of staff can be integrated with the organizations goals and purposes. This process first occurs on the intraorganizational level and then must be applied to the interorganizational arena where cross training takes place. Interorganizational in-service cross training becomes more complicated, since the goals and purposes of *two* organizations have to be integrated and the abilities and skills of each staff considered.

In the case situation, it might have been useful for the family agency to develop cross training with the CMHC so that the staffs from both of these organizations could become more familiar with each other's service operations. This can be a first step in developing better service coordination.

From the above discussion of the functions of the resource coordination unit, it must be evident that considerable responsibility is lodged in this organizational unit. Negotiating affiliation and liaisonship agreements requires having substantial authority to interact with administrators in other agencies. Therefore, it is crucial that the agency administrator provide the sanction and support needed by the resource coordination unit to engage in the negotiation of interagency agreements. Having discussed the administrative support for resource coordination, we now proceed to the role of the community planner in facilitating community resource coordination.

Community Level: Community Planning

Community planners can facilitate community resource coordination through activities in three areas: (1) diagnosing the local service-delivery system; (2) facilitating interagency coordination; and (3) monitoring resource coordination.

Diagnosing the Service-Delivery System

As we indicated above, assessment of the local delivery system can be done by the resource coordination unit. Planning on the community level, however, provides an opportunity for a more comprehensive approach to community assessment. This comprehensive approach requires detailed information on the nature of the local service-delivery system. The following is a model for an integrated human service-delivery system that a community planner can use as a tool for diagnosing the strengths and weaknesses of a particular system and taking actions to obtain more effective community resource coordination. Such community analysis will facilitate *community need assessment.*

Components of an Integrated Service-Delivery System

Aiken et al. (1975) suggest that at least four elements must be coordinated in a fully integrated service-delivery system: (1) programs and services; (2) resources; (3) clients; and (4) information. Each of these is an important and essential ingredient in any fully integrated service delivery system and the coordination of any one of these components does not necessarily imply the coordination of another.

Linkages among these four elements can be created by drawing upon three principles of coordination: (1) comprehensiveness, (2) compatibility, and (3) cooperation (Aiken et al. 1975:10-15). *Comprehensiveness* refers to whether a system has all of the resources and programs necessary to serve users adequately. For example, a comprehensive service system to enable the severely disabled to live in the community should have programs to meet essential needs such as food, shelter, employment, training, and health care. *Compatibility* assumes the proper linkage and sequencing of programs so that service consumers get services when they need them. Survival needs such as money and housing should have higher priority than meeting service users' social emotional needs (Maslow 1970).

Cooperation includes both a behavioral and an attitudinal component (e.g., common effort and willingness to work together). This will depend on "mutual understanding, minimum shared goals and values, and ability to work together on a common task" (Aiken et al. 1975:9). As previously indicated, a fully coordinated system needs to integrate programs, resources, service consumers, and information with the three principles of comprehensiveness, compatibility, and cooperation. The linking of the four elements and three principles will be illustrated by use of the case situation.

Program Coordination

Program coordination assumes the existence of *comprehensive* services (i.e., all the necessary services must be available). In the case, comprehensive programming was not available because of the absence of housing services. Program coordination also requires *compatible* services; to allow for the proper linking and sequencing of services. As indicated previously, sequencing of services depends on a determination of service priorities. In the case example, survival needs such as housing and money would receive attention before other service needs. Finally, effective programming requires that professionals have *cooperative* working relationships. In the case, successful cooperation was diminished by the lack of common goals between the staff of the FSSA and the CMHC.

Resource Coordination

Effective service also requires the coordination of resources such as funding, staff, facilities, power, legitimation, etc. Since a *comprehensive* system of funding usually does not exist, gaps in financial resources should be filled by more efficient use of existing resources, such as the sharing and exchange of staff, facilities, etc. In the case situation, the assumption by the Family Service Agency of case coordination for discharged mental patients by the FSSA is an example of resource sharing between two agencies. Allocation of resources in a manner that is *compatible* with service user need insures that service priorities favor those service consumers with the most urgent needs. In the case, priority would be given to severely mentally disabled service users. Resources at the CMHC should be reallocated from the less-disabled service consumers to the more severely mentally ill. This might require the replacement of therapeutically trained staff with practitioners trained in psychosocial rehabilitation (Anthony, Cohen, and Nemec 1987). *Cooperation* among those who control resources requires collaboration between funding authorities. This can be done on the community level through planning and allocating agencies, assuming they are the channel through which funds are distributed in the community. In the case situation, the community planning agency could have assumed such a role.

Service User Coordination

Coordination of service consumers assures that all eligible service users are served (*comprehensiveness*). In the case situation, all the patients from the mental hospital had access to case coordination services through the FSSA. *Compatible* services for consumers requires the proper sequencing of these programs. In the case situation, the case coordinator should develop plans for each service user to insure that services are provided when needed. For example, short-term emergency services in a protective setting would be followed by extended care in a more normalized setting in the community. *Cooperative* activities would include some means for service-user representatives to give feedback to the service providers. In the case, a service-consumer advocate organization, such as one representing the families of the mentally ill, could be used to provide this feedback.

Coordination of Information

Lastly, the coordination of service user information requires a *comprehensive* record-keeping system where information about services and service consumer needs (compatibility) is integrated with continuous feedback from the service users to achieve effective operation of the system (cooperation). Automated information systems are essential for integrated case management (Ezell and Patti 1990:30). In the case situation, this type of information system should be the responsibility of the community planning agency.

Aiken et al. (1975:16) suggest that these elements are coordinated by different levels of the service system: resources at the policy level; programs at the community planning level; service consumers at the worker and organizational level; and information at all three levels. They argue that an optimal service-delivery system requires coordination on all three levels.

If one were to apply the above criteria to the case situation, it would be evident that there are deficiencies in the system of care for the severely mentally ill. The above model provides an *ideal* that can be used by the administrator, planner, and policy analyst to loate system weaknesses and can assist efforts to develop a more integrated and functional service-delivery system.

Several characteristics of the local delivery system have been identified as relevant to the diagnosis of resource coordination problems (Beatrice 1981). A characteristic related to comprehensiveness is whether there is bias in the system (e.g., favoring institutional over home care). This kind of bias in the medical-care system can be obviated by having hospitals serve as entry points into a community-care system (Netting and Williams 1989). Also associated with system comprehensiveness is the extent of duplication and overlapping of services, as well as the quality of the services provided.

A second characteristic of the local service-delivery system that could present problems for resource coordinators is the provider's power to resist resource coordinator controls. This power involves the control of critical resources: service users, information, and funding. A centralized system with a single point of entry would minimize the power of the providers to resist resource coordinator controls. Similarly, the control of funding by the resource coordinator will have an influence on his or her capacity to change providers' behavior (Baxter et al. 1983:27). The power of the resource coordinator to use financial incentives and sanctions such as cost controls on services could be used to fill in gaps in services. In the case situation, it may have been possible for the case coordinator to influence the CMHC to provide adequate service if financial incentives were available.

The community planner's assessment of the nature of the service-delivery system can provide the community resource case coordinator (Lauffer 1978:191-193) with information that will enable him or her to appreciate the opportunities and/or constraints operating on his or her actions. This assessment can also provide the information needed to facilitate better interagency service coordination—the second function that is performed by the community planner.

Facilitating Interagency Coordination

Community planners can facilitate interagency coordination by using negotiating skills to mediate interorganizational conflict and competition and facilitate agency awareness of interdependence (Lauffer 1978:76).

Interorganizational conflict and competition is often related to problems in achieving domain consensus between agencies. Domain consensus involves settlement of boundary (turf) disputes and agreement over the way resources are divided (Austin 1981). Community planners can mediate between agencies to help them obtain agreements on who will provide which kinds of services to what types of service users. These agreements can be formalized in the form of affiliation and liaisonship contracts.

Interorganizational coordination can also be furthered by community planners through their role of facilitating agency awareness of interdependence. Since agency interdependency is related to shared goals and opportunities for the exchange of resources, the community planner should first determine whether in fact these two preconditions for coordination exist. If they do, the planner can then make this information visible to the administrators of the respective agencies, the first step in helping them to understand that it would be to their mutual benefit to develop a cooperative relationship. In the analysis of the barriers to coordination, the planner needs to differentiate between the influence of economic, political; and psychological factors (Neugeboren 1991:220-222); professional ideologies; service consumers' interests; resource controllers' values; and multiple governmental auspices (Aiken et al. 1975:19-24; Lauffer 1978:214-218).

In the case, the planner would have to take into account the political influence of the CMHC board, the service user's interests, and the funding authority's expectations before attempting to facilitate interorganizational coordination. He might have helped the CMHC and the FSSA by making them aware of their interdependencies, such as their sharing of goals. In this situation the planner should be sensitive to the possibility that there might be ideological barriers preventing coordination between the two agencies. The planner would then have to develop strategies to avoid a direct confrontation between the psychologically oriented CMHC staff and the socially oriented FSSA staff. Negotiating skills would be used to focus on areas of common self-interest, rather than on differences in philosophy that cannot be negotiated.

Community planners can also facilitate interagency coordination through fiscal mechanisms such as purchase of services, joint budgeting, and joint funding (Lauffer 1978:188-191). In the case, the planner might use joint funding of the CMHC and the FSSA to facilitate cooperation between these two organizations.

Monitoring Resource Coordination

Planning and allocating agencies are responsible for monitoring service delivery programs that they fund (Lauffer 1978:81-83). The efficiency and effectiveness of community resource coordination can be determined by using the criteria discussed above as evidence that agencies are developing arrangements to work together more cooperatively.

In the case situation, the community planner performed this monitoring function through an assessment that showed that there were gaps in treatment services for the severely mentally ill. He also discovered that there were alternative programs available (those for the developmentally disabled and physically handicapped) that would also be appropriate for the severely mentally ill.

We have discussed how administrators and planners can create links with the resource coordinator role and function. Now we will show how the role of the policy analyst is related to community resource coordination.

Societal Level: Policy Analysis

Social policy analysts are responsible for formulating new policies or modifying existing policies to achieve better coordination and integration of services (Jansson 1984:113-114). *Goal clarification,* which assesses the relationship between the means and ends of human service programs, determines whether policies favoring institutional over integrated community-based programs better serve the needs of the severely disabled. Policies that foster service duplication and fragmentation may necessitate a modification in policies governing *strategies* for achieving goals (Jansson 1984:19). More-unified structures may be required to solve the problem of service fragmentation. However, although service integration (i.e., placement of programs under a single administrative authority) has been successfully introduced in Europe, this has not widely been the case in the United States, where categorical funding with specialized constituencies is a constraining factor (Morris and Lescohier 1978). Given the difficulties of achieving service integration, policy analysts should examine the potential for service coordination. Policies that foster interorganizational cooperation may be required so as to provide for coordination between autonomous agencies. For example, funding authorities could require inter-agency affiliation agreements as a precondition for grants. Legislation could promote integration rather than separation of services. For example, departments of drug and alcohol abuse could be combined into a department for substance abuse.

Policy analysts also have to consider the possibility that the defects in the service-delivery system stem not from lack of coordination of existing resources, but from a *deficiency* or gap in these resources (Aiken et al. 1975:6) If resource deficiency is the problem, then policy analysts should rectify this through the formulation of policies that add programs to fill in the gaps. In the case example, the lack of sheltered housing was a resource deficiency that could be rectified by the policy analyst through the formulation of legislation to remedy this defect. This deficiency was noticed by the community resource case coordinator and communicated to the administrator, who in turn made this information available to the community planner. He should further document the need and the deficiency and provide the information to the policy analyst. This process has been termed coordination by feedback (March and Simon 1958).

SUMMARY

Community resource coordination at the macro level is an integral part of a comprehensive system for case coordination. It provides the structural support required for an effective system of interagency cooperation and coordination.

Macro organizational-level intervention (administration) was illustrated with the function of the resource coordination unit. Macro community-level intervention (community planning) included the functions of diagnosing the service-delivery system, facilitating interagency cooperation, and monitoring. Macro societal-level (intervention social policy analysis) involved formulation of new policies and modification of existing policies in order to enhance service coordination and/or integration.

STUDY QUESTIONS

1. You are the FSSA administrator mentioned in the case. Your staff informs you that the CMHC is reluctant to serve the severely mentally ill service consumers who are being seen in your agency. What steps would you take to determine if there is a basis for interagency collaboration between your agency and the CMHC? What skills would you use?

2. Think about an agency with which you are familiar. Identify its organizational set by determining who refers service users to this agency and where this agency sends their service consumers. What are the implications of these referral patterns for interagency relations?

3. Identify a situation where two agencies are in conflict. Analyze the basis of this conflict in terms of similarity or differences in goals. Determine whether there is any basis for cooperation between these two agencies in terms of resource dependency.

4. You are director of the resource coordination unit of the FSSA. Develop a plan for initiation of an interagency agreement between your agency and a program for the developmentally disabled for service for the provision of the severely mentally ill. What skills would you need to implement this plan?

5. You are a community planner. What would you do to deal with the interagency conflict between the FSSA and the CMHC? What skills would you use?

6. You are a community planner diagnosing the adequacy of the service-delivery system in your community. What elements and principles would you need to understand to do a comprehensive assessment of the extent to which services are coordinated?

7. You are a policy analyst. Determine what modifications in social policy may be required to facilitate interagency coordination for the severely mentally ill. Apply the policy framework discussed in Chapter 2.

Chapter 6

SOCIAL SUPPORT
ON THE MICRO LEVEL

Social Support
on the Micro Level

I.   Introduction
II.   Case: Frail Elderly
     A. Case Goals and Interventions
        1. Obtain Aid from Neighbors
        2. Coordination of Health-Care Services
        3. Help Mrs. S Cope with Her Husband's Death
        4. Help Resolve the Mother-Daughter Conflict
III. Issues
     A. Costs vs. Benefits of Social Support
     B. Opportunities and Constraints of Integrating Formal and Informal Care Systems
     C. Social Support and Prevention of Social Problems
IV. Definitions
     A. Social Support
        1. Mutual Aid
        2. Self-Help
        3. Support Systems
V.   Targets of Social Support
     A. Service Users
     B. Informal Caregivers
     C. Formal Caregivers
     D. Community At Large
VI. Interventions
     A. Organizational Arena: Direct Practice
        1. Preparatory Interventions
           a. Assessment
           b. Screening
           c. Anticipatory Guidance

INTRODUCTION

Human service professionals, prompted by evidence that social isolation is an important contributor to individual and family dysfunction (Garbarino 1977; Rothman 1994:106) have shown increasing interest in social support interventions for dealing with social problems. One indication of this trend is the two-dozen articles on social networks and social support published in social work journals during the years 1977 to 1985 (Specht 1988:184). This activity reflects a departure from the traditional people-changing technologies incorporated in the methods of casework, group work, and community organization (Specht 1988:175), toward intervention strategies that focus on environmental change.

This chapter is devoted to a discussion of social support on the micro level in the organizational and community arenas, particularly the functions of direct-service and community organizations. Macro level support interventions of the administrator, planner, and policy analyst, will be discussed in Chapter 7. Although the micro and macro levels of intervention are dealt with separately, effective practice requires an understanding of both levels.

This chapter begins with a case description that illustrates the use of social support as a direct-practice intervention with an elderly person. This case will be referred to throughout the chapter to indicate how the principles and interventions of social support are relevant in a practice situation and how intervention skills discussed in Chapter 2 are also used for this purpose. The section on definitions of social support includes a look at the types and targets of this human service technology. Micro level interventions in the organizational and community practice arenas are then discussed. Specific study questions conclude the chapter.

CASE: FRAIL ELDERLY

Mrs. S is a 75-year-old woman who recently became widowed. She had been married for 55 years and has two children, a 50-year-old daughter who is married with no children, and a 40-year-old son married with two children, ages 15 and 10. Mrs. S lives alone in an apartment in an urban area. Her sole income is from social security.

She socializes with neighbors in the apartment house, but does not have any close relationships. Mrs. S' daughter lives about ten blocks from her mother's home. She works full time and visits her mother in the evenings and on weekends. The son, who resides in another state, visits with the family about once a month.

After Mrs. S' husband died she became depressed and developed health problems, including arthritis, heart problems, symptoms of paranoia, and a thyroid condition. She had separate physicians for each of her health problems and received different medications for each condition. There was little coordination of her health care. Up until her husband's death, Mrs. S continued to function well in the performance of household duties, including taking care of her husband through a long illness that preceded his death. Throughout her adult life, Mrs. S was a very independent person who was able to fulfill her responsibilities without the help of others.

Her dominant personality generated conflict with her daughter and son-in-law. As Mrs. S became more disabled by arthritis, she turned more and more to her daughter for help with shopping, transportation to doctors, cooking, and other household chores. The power struggle between mother and daughter increased as the latter gained dominance because of the mother's dependency. Through the course of years, the son freed himself from the mother's influence by living in another state, where he was involved with his own family and career. Mrs. S expressed positive feelings about her son and was proud of his success in his profession.

The son and daughter became increasingly concerned about their mother's inability to care for herself, as well as for her safety. There were several incidents where Mrs. S fell in her apartment and was unable to get up because of the arthritis. Her inability to walk prevented her from leaving the apartment and led to her social isolation. The mother was examined by a neurologist to determine the reason for her falls, but no definitive cause was found. Mrs. S also developed paranoid mental symptoms. She was seen by a psychiatrist, who prescribed antipsychotic medication. The daughter thought that she might have to place her mother in a protective setting, such as a nursing home.

The daughter, who bore the brunt of the responsibility for the mother's care, became increasingly distressed and sought help from a local family-service agency. They assigned a social worker who met with Mrs. S and the daughter and son.

Case Goals and Interventions

The social worker developed the following goals and interventions related to social support:

1. Facilitate the mother's receiving emergency aid from neighbors.
2. Coordinate health care services.
3. Help Mrs. S' cope with her husbands death.
4. Help resolve the mother-daughter conflict.

Obtain Aid from Neighbors

The social worker first did an evaluation of the neighborhood where Mrs. S resided. She discovered that an informal helping system existed among the residents in this apartment house. Since many of these residents were elderly women living alone, they turned to each other for help when they were temporarily incapacitated by illnesses. She also determined that the residents came from the same ethnic group and had lived in the area for many years. Although the neighbors did not become closely involved with each other, they assisted each other with such tasks as food shopping.

The worker dealt with the problem of Mrs. S falling by suggesting that emergency help could be provided by neighbors. A plan was developed for her to use an emergency alarm device, which consisted of a pendant with a call button worn around the neck. When pressed, it alerted an emergency phone service that phoned one or more of the neighbors. The neighbor would then have the superintendent of the building let her into Mrs. S' apartment to determine the problem.

The staffperson also asked Mrs. S which neighbors had been helpful. The worker discovered that the neighbor living in the apartment door had assisted Mrs. S with her shopping. With Mrs. S' permission, the worker enlisted the aid of Mrs. S' neighbors. One important objective was to have the neighbors visit Mrs. S in her apartment to monitor how she was doing and to arrange for their help in an emergency. The social worker approached the neighbors by meeting with them where they congregated in front of the house.

The worker explained the situation to the neighbors and they discussed the different ways that they could offer help. Initially, these neighbors were somewhat hesitant to become involved. They perceived the social worker as someone who dealt with "problems," rather than such normal situations as a neighbor needing a helping hand. Aware of the neighbors' orientation, the social worker discussed Mr. S' situation as something that could happen to anyone. They indeed recognized that there were other people in the apartment house who were in a somewhat similar situation. The worker also decided that it would be useful to contact a community organizer who worked on the local Citizen's Committee for the Elderly for assistance.

The community organizer discovered that one of the neighbors was very active in helping others. In their discussions, the worker helped the neighbor to see how the plan for dealing with emergencies for Mrs. S could also be applied to other elderly people in the apartment house. A meeting was held where the community organizer explained the medical alarm system to the tenants, which helped generate more mutual helping among the tenants in the building.

The community organizer also become aware in her work with disabled elderly that there was a need for a more organized system of neighbors helping each other in times of emergency. She contacted current and past service consumers in the neighborhood who had a need for an emergency alarm service like the one developed for Mrs. S. They were invited to a community meeting where they decided to organize a self-help group called Medical Alert, in which neighbors would be available to assist each other in times of emergency. The community organizer provided assistance to this group to help it become formally organized. Eventually, the group successfully petitioned the government social-services agency to establish a fund to pay the rent on medical alarms for disabled persons.

Coordination of Health-Care Services

Since Mrs. S was being seen by several doctors, there was a need to coordinate their services. One problem was the fact that Mrs. S' multiple medications were not being monitored for possible negative interactions. There was a possibility that the falls and the psychological symptoms were due to overmedication. The social worker consulted with an internist who was seeing Mrs. S and he found that several of the drugs could interact negatively and could produce the falling and psychological symptoms. The internist took on the responsibility of coordinating Mrs. S' medication with the other physicians. At the social worker's suggestion, he enlisted the pharmacist's cooperation in the future monitoring of the drugs being prescribed. As a result of these efforts, the psychological symptoms and falling decreased.

The worker also was aware that this problem of overmedication due to lack of coordinated health services was common among the service users in her caseload. She contacted the community organizer, who subsequently became involved in working with the community to solve this serious problem. She met with informal leaders of the community and encouraged them to assume leadership of a community effort to resolve this problem of lack of coordination of drug treatment of the elderly.

These leaders arranged for a meeting of formal and informal community leaders to discuss this problem. In addition to the informal leaders, representatives from the local senior citizen center, the medical and pharmaceutical societies, and the community social-planning agency were invited to this meeting. The problem of overmedication was discussed, and various solutions proposed, and committees organized to implement these solutions. A feasible plan was developed to coordinate medication through a cooperative effort of the physicians and pharmacies, which included the installation of a computer system in the pharmacies that alerted the pharmacist when a new drug that was prescribed had the potential for negative drug interactions. This successful community organization effort laid the groundwork for the creation of an ongoing community organization that took responsibility for addressing various community problems and developing solutions to them.

Help Mrs. S Cope with Her Husband's Death

The social worker attempted to counsel Mrs. S regarding her depression over her husband's death. Mrs. S was very reluctant to admit being depressed, saying that she was glad that his suffering was over. The worker decided that a referral to a "Widowed Persons" self-help group was indicated. This group met at the local senior citizen center. Mrs. S was reluctant to attend the group because she could not see how it would help her medical problems. Also, Mrs. S was not a "joiner"–she had never participated actively in groups. Since she had a medical orientation to her problems, the social worker sought the doctor's help in persuading Mrs. S to attend a meeting of the self-help group. The doctor initially resisted the suggestion that Mrs. S could benefit from participation in a self help group, because he also saw her problems as primarily medical. The social worker overcame his objections by giving him an article from a medical journal that showed how social support was useful in the treatment of medical problems.

Since Mrs. S had expressed positive feelings about her son, the social worker also enlisted his support in encouraging his mother to attend the self-help group. The worker was careful not to have the daughter involved in pressuring the mother to go to the self-help group, since their relationship was problematic.

Because Mrs. S was still ambivalent about attending the self-help group, a member of this group visited Mrs. S and persuaded her to come to one meeting. This woman was also recently widowed and explained to Mrs. S how the people in the group helped each other. The social worker arranged transportation for Mrs. S and a recently widowed neighbor who was interested in joining the group. Mrs. S attended several meetings and discovered much similarity between herself and other group members in their feelings about their husbands' deaths.

As a result, Mrs. S' depression lifted, with a corresponding diminishment in arthritis symptoms. Another consequence of her attendance at the widow's group was her participation in social activities at the center that reduced her social isolation.

Help Resolve the Mother-Daughter Conflict

The social worker concluded from talking with the daughter that she was conflicted over the problem of balancing her responsibility for her mother and her own personal needs. Referral to a mutual aid group of children of aged parents was made. The daughter also found that sharing with others in a similar situation as herself helped to relieve her anxiety and conflict regarding her responsibilities toward her mother. In addition, she learned about the problems that widows experience when their partners died, which helped her understand better how her father's death was affecting her mother. Her tension and the accompanying nervousness that caused sleeping difficulties lessened. The mother's involvement in the senior citizen center and the daughter's participation in a self-help group helped to decrease the conflict between them.

ISSUES

In light of the positive effects of informal social support, the question is how can formal service programs utilize this knowledge to enhance their effectiveness in service provision and prevention? What are the limitations of social support and what inhibits micro and macro practitioners from incorporating it in the human services? What are the opportunities and constraints of integrating formal and informal care systems? Also, can social support intervention be an effective strategy to prevent social problems? These questions will be addressed in this section.

Costs vs. Benefits of Social Support

Caution is being urged on the wholesale introduction of social support as a major intervention strategy in the human services. There is concern that professional interventions in informal support systems can be overly intrusive and controlling, and may promote dependency. Also, the need to rely on family members who suffer from similar social problems or on neighbors who view the individual's behavior as deviancy may increase rather than lessen the stress (Gottlieb 1983:63). Professional intervention into informal care networks may reduce the motivation of an informal helper to continue to provide support (Gottlieb 1983:116).

A historical perspective makes us aware that the use of lay support is really not a new phenomenon. Social support and the use of informal helping systems have roots in the early history of social work, such as in the charity societies and the settlement houses that used lay volunteers to provide services. A renewed partnership between professionals and laypersons to help people deal with problems of daily living is evident in studies of practice in the United States (Froland et al. 1981:55) and abroad (Pancoast, Parker, and Froland 1983).

Critics have questioned the effectiveness of this type of intervention (Di Matteo and Hays 1981:121; Levy 1982:155-172). However, the picture is mixed, since there is evidence also of positive outcomes produced by the integration of programs of formal and informal support. In a study of 30 agencies, positive outcomes included "increased accessibility and responsiveness of services; increased cost efficiency and use of informal resources; reduction in institutionalization of clients; increased local participation and control in service delivery" (Froland et al. 1981:85-108).

Critics are concerned that a social support service-delivery policy will be used merely for purposes of cost containment. The interest in voluntarism dominant under the Reagan administration has led to the use of nongovernmental support as an excuse for diminished public funding of services (Gottlieb 1983:216-217; Hopps 1986:419; Schilling, Schinke, and Weatherly 1988: Specht 1988:182-183).

Changing demographic trends also seem to indicate decreasing potential for social support. The diminished relevance of the extended family with increased geographic mobility and the changing role of women suggests a reduction in the traditional sources of social support (Schilling 1988:6-7). If we accept the value of social support interventions, this diminution in traditional social support networks should obligate us to seek alternate sources of social support. This loss of "personal communities" requires other social buffers for dealing with the problems of living (Gottlieb 1983:217-218). Human-service professionals are broadening their view of personal problems and seeing them within a community and situational "context" (Anthony 1979:27; Froland et al. 1981:121-150). The beliefs that the *gemeinschaft* (Tonnies 1957), or informal community, is no longer applicable in an urban society, or that we have romanticized the idea of community because we thought we had lost it (Panzetta 1971:1-19), are being questioned. The community is viewed in broader terms: "it is more than the geographic unit in which we practice: it is a unit of social structure that brings meaning and sense of coherence to people's lives" (Gottlieb 1983:219). Social networks are an important factor in defining problems, providing help, influencing what kinds of help will be accepted, and aiding the way people adjust to acute and chronic problems (Froland et. al 1981:21).

Questions have also been raised about the appropriateness of social support for lower-income (Auslander and Litwin 1988) and pathological and deviant individuals. Since informal care is based on reciprocity in helping, and a certain level of social competence is a precondition for access to social support (Gottlieb 1983: 79-80), it is believed that this intervention strategy is more relevant for stable and affluent populations (Judge and Smith 1983). On the other hand, self help groups have been developed successfully for less-functional populations such as the chronically mentally ill (Froland et al. 1981:74-75) and the homeless (Marin and Vacha 1994). Stimulus for the use of social support interventions for the chronically mentally ill has come from deinstitutionalization policies result in large numbers of disabled persons being discharged into the community. Support strategies are viewed as a particularly appropriate way to enable the mentally ill (Salem, Seiderman, and Rappaport 1988), the developmentally and physically disabled, children, youth and families, elderly, and low-income families (Froland 1981:58) with long-term disabilities to be able to live and adjust in the community.

Given the mixed picture of the effectiveness of social support and the potential for adverse effects, one must ask whether scarce resources should be shifted from the more-traditional services to the social support modality. We need to temper our criticism of this more recent mode of intervention with the realization that the outcomes of the more-traditional services are also somewhat mixed (Fischer 1973; Reid and Hanrahan 1982; Rubin 1985). It would be unfortunate to use a higher standard to evaluate a new intervention than was the case with the more established ones. We should not allow our ideological biases and vested interests in the status quo to deter efforts to experiment with this new intervention, even if it means that other service methods are given a lower priority.

Opportunities and Constraints of Integrating Formal and Informal Care Systems

A central issue related to the integration of formal and informal care systems is the effect of professional involvement in the informal care system. Would attempts of professionals to combine their efforts with those of lay helpers diminish the normative orientation of these persons that is the unique basis of their support? If this is so, then would it not be better for these two systems of care to remain separate? It has been suggested that there may be a lack of congruency between professional and nonprofessional helping, due to differences in modes of functioning, values, and power. Lay knowledge, which is based on individual or shared experience, contrasts with professional technical knowledge derived from science and research (Lauffer 1984:90). For example, the professional tends to stress personality in contrast to the nonprofessional stress on environment (Gottlieb 1983:27). Do the differences in the social characteristics of professional and nonprofessional helpers (Mechanic 1980:159) and the nature of professional training (Specht 1988:166) work to undermine the effectiveness of informal support? Does the individual orientation in which human service professionals are trained, and the bureaucratic structures within which they work, conflict with the communal basis of informal support systems (Specht 1988:166; Litwak and Meyer 1966)? Will professional cooperation with informal systems of care result in their "annexation" and the loss of their unique contributions? Professions prefer linking roles as consultants, facilitators, speakers and organizers (Toseland and Hacker 1985), while mutual-aid group members desire a more egalitarian relationship (Kurtz 1984).

Do formal agencies need the help of informal caregivers to facilitate their efforts? Conversely, are resources from the formal care system needed to bolster the efforts of informal helpers, particularly in long-term disability situations?

The above potential issues of collaboration between the formal and informal care systems suggest that professionals should redefine their roles so that their efforts complement rather than conflict with the roles performed by the informal system (Gottlieb 1983:218-219). The nature of these new professional roles will be discussed below in the section on practice interventions. In the case situation, the worker successfully linked with a self-help group for Mrs. S and her daughter.

Social Support and Prevention of Social Problems

The research on the buffering effects of social support suggests the potential use of this type of intervention for preventive purposes (Ballew 1985). Thus, stress-reducing interventions into such crisis situations as unemployment, bereavement, retirement, disability, and remarriage have been found to prevent the development of illness (Gottlieb 1983:67-106). The positive effects of social support were demonstrated in an experimental study of the use of the *"doula"* (a supportive companion for women in childbirth) in Guatemala. The doula, an untrained laywoman previously unknown to the expectant mother, provided support in the form of physical contact, dialogue, and simple companionship from the point of admission until delivery. Comparison of experimental and control groups found that the former had 50 percent fewer serious complications in delivery (Sosa et al. 1980).

A prevention-related question on that has been raised about those programs in general is whether scarce resources should be diverted from service to persons with serious disabilities (e.g., mentally ill) to those who are not suffering. The value of preventive interventions is complicated by the difficulty of making accurate predictions of the consequences of interventions vs. noninterventions (Garbarino 1980; Mechanic 1980:162; Neugeboren 1991:12-13). However, substantial evidence that social support can prevent illness suggests that it may be fruitful to invest resources in this intervention area.

DEFINITIONS

This section on the definition of social support first presents a generic definition that includes both formal professional and informal lay support. Mutual aid, self-help, and support systems are then discussed as particular kinds of social support. Social support is then described more specifically in terms of four targets: service consumers, informal caregivers, formal caregivers, and the community at large.

Social Support

Gottlieb defines social support in terms of the roles of informal care givers (Gottlieb 1983:28-29). We expand his formulation to include formal agency caregivers in order to make it a more generic activity and arrive at the following definition: social support involves verbal and/or nonverbal information or advice, tangible aid, or action provided by social intimates and/or professional caregivers that has beneficial emotional or behavioral effects on the recipient.

This expansion of the definition of social support is not meant to diminish the importance of the mutuality involved in peer support. Including professional support as part of the definition emphasizes the potential for formal caregivers to have a role in the provision of social support. Evidence indicates equal effectiveness of peer-led and professional-led support groups (Toseland, Rossiter, and Labreque 1989). A distinction is made, however, between the traditional "treatment" roles assumed by professionals and that of a social support role (Schopler and Galinsky 1993).

Social support, whether provided by peers or professionals, stresses the environmental support of natural helping networks. Professional social support facilitates the effective operation of the natural lay system of support. The professional role is directed at environment-changing goals, rather than therapeutic people-changing goals. Social support therefore has a "normative" emphasis that views people's difficulties as "problems of living" (Mechanic 1980:5) and "life crises," rather than in "pathological" or "sickness" terms. Social support is assumed to be a natural and ongoing process that is intrinsic to coping with problems of daily life. Therefore, it does not view interdependency negatively, but rather as a natural and inevitable part of social life resulting in the mutual exchange of resources.

This is shown in our case situation. The social worker, in addition to facilitating aid from the informal support system (Mrs. S' neighbors) also helped bolster the operation of this system by facilitating mutual aid in the medical alarm system. She also emphasized the normative aspect of Mrs. S' difficulties of old age.

The contribution of nonprofessional helping, which is intrinsic to social support, differs from that of professional service and has major advantages by virtue of:

(a) its natural accessibility; (b) its congruence with local norms about when and how support ought to be expressed; (c) its rootedness in long-standing peer relationships; (d) its variability, ranging from the provision of tangible goods and services to simple companionship; and (e) its freedom from financial and psychological (stigma) costs incurred when professional resources are used. (Gottlieb 1983:27)

The professional, in addressing the task of facilitating informal support, should be cognizant of the above major differences between formal and informal helping.

In the case situation, the advantages of the informal helping system of Mrs. S' neighbors were evident. Its accessibility was particularly important in dealing with the problem of emergencies that might arise because of Mrs. S' falling and for which she might require immediate help.

Mutual Aid

Froland et al. (1981:72) defines mutual aid as "actual or potential relationships among a set of individuals who come together because they have experienced similar problems, face common tasks, or have compatible interests or abilities." As is generally true for self-help, mutual aid encourages normalization and social integration and a sense of confidence in sharing problems and helping others. Mutual aid in times of crisis differs substantively from individual crisis intervention (Lindemann 1944; Caplan 1964), in that the former relies heavily on peer support and leadership, utilizing the process of social comparison. Through this process, people receive support through the reassurance that others in similar environmental situations experience parallel difficulties.

By witnessing other ways of overcoming similar difficulties, people learn to appreciate the healing effects of time. Group sharing counteracts feelings of isolation and uniqueness that increase stress (Gottlieb 1983:70). Since mutual aid involves reciprocity in relationships and requires a level of motivation necessary to self-initiation, it is less feasible with individuals who are socially limited (e.g., isolated elderly, developmentally disabled, mentally ill). For these kinds of persons, self-help is a more appropriate intervention. The principle of reciprocity is illustrated in the case in the manner in which this population of elderly women living alone in their apartments dealt with their need for short-term assistance.

Self-Help

Self-help is similar to mutual aid, but is more formally organized and structured. Thus, self-help groups have explicit charters, a specific ideology, and a standardized program (Gottlieb 1983:51–52) that is under the auspice of formal agencies. While mutual aid involves naturally formed groups, self-help is more formally organized (e.g., Alcoholics Anonymous). Formally organized self-help groups have the advantage of providing useful information, such as members' experience with service providers, which can be used to evaluate their services. Data can also be made available on the latest service innovations (e.g., recently developed successful drug treatments). Self-help groups also view their goals as empowerment on an individual, organizational, and societal level (Segal, Silverman, and Temkon 1993).

The case situation illustrated a principle that is basic to both mutual aid and self-help: that people having similar situational problems can share and obtain social support through a process of social comparison. This was evident in the Widowed Persons self-help group attended by Mrs. S, as well as in the group for children with elderly parents attended by the daughter.

Support Systems

Support systems involve formal agencies, informal family, and neighborhood caregivers (i.e., a combination of both formal and informal systems). Agency support systems involve the coordination of an array of services that provide support to specific service consumers (e.g., community support systems for the developmentally disabled) (Stein 1979). A detailed discussion of community resource coordination, which is the basis for formal agency support systems, was included in Chapters 3 and 4.

Informal support systems have been termed "natural helping networks" and are neighborhood-based (Collins and Pancoast 1976). Natural helping networks rely on network members who, because of residential proximity can exchange needed services, goods, and emotional support with minimum reliance on professionals.

Interweaving of formal and informal care systems involves a partnership of the community and the social-service system. It starts from a

> Perspective of the community or locality as a caregiving system by seeking to reinforce and optimize existing resources and creating resources to fill gaps in provision . . . view the entire community as both needing and offering support . . .
> Interweaving is not shifting responsibility from formal to informal services. Neither is about co-opting and colonizing informal systems or about superimposing existing packages of care on the community. (Grant and Wenger 1983:48)

The interweaving of formal and informal care systems was evident in the case example. The existing informal care system of the neighbors in the apartment house was linked with services of a local family-service agency, resulting in an enhancement of both systems.

TARGETS OF SOCIAL SUPPORT

There are five targets toward which social support activities can be directed: service users, informal caregivers, formal caregivers, and the community at large.

Service Users

The discussion of service consumers as a target for social support, will begin with an exploration of their needs during life crises, followed by a discussion of types of program interventions.

The discussion of social support in life crises will focus on the effects of stress in two areas: illness experience and care of the elderly.

Six kinds of threats have been associated with *illness experience*: (1) threats to life; (2) threats to bodily integrity and comfort; (3) threats to self-concept and future plans; (4) threats to emotional equilibrium;

(5) threats to fulfillment of customary roles; and (6) threats associated with the demands of adjusting to a new physical or social environment (Cohen and Lazarus 1979). Support groups were found to be helpful in dealing with these consequences associated with such illnesses as heart disease and breast cancer (Gottlieb 1983:151-160). Another area in which social support has been found useful is stress reduction in the elderly.

In the case example, it is evident that Mrs. S was undergoing a life crisis with various threats as a result of her husband's death. She experienced a threat to her self-concept in that she lost her autonomy and became dependent on others, in contrast to her previous ability to be in control of her life situation. Related to this was her loss of her role as wife and caretaker, a role which had helped her feel needed and gave her a purpose.

Informal Caregivers

In general, there are three sources of informal support available: family, friends, and neighbors and others. Each of these sources of support serves a different purpose (Richardson, Graham, and Shelton 1989). Family support is turned to in times of illness and financial adversity. Families can provide concrete support such as housing to prevent or postpone institutionalization (Froland et al. 1981:189-191). Friends provide support that builds life satisfaction and morale. Neighbors can provide information about local services and can respond to time-limited emergency needs. Four types of support (friendship and socialization; emotional support; practical assistance; guidance and advice) have been included in a worksheet used to determine need and availability of social support (Rothman 1994:165). In the case, Mrs. S received support from her family regarding her illness and from neighbors in emergency situations.

Informal caregivers include not only the family, friends, and neighbors, but also others, such as bartenders, beauticians, foremen, and so forth. However, the positive effects of caregiver support on the chronically disabled are most evident in family support groups (Toseland et al. 1990; Toseland 1990).

In environmental practice, the *family* is an important social resource (Specht 1988:167). In the area of mental illness, traditional treatment often sees the family as contributing to the individual's problems. In contrast, environmental practice operates on the premise that there is little scientific basis to suggest that psychiatric disorder is caused by childhood upbringing or family interactions (Mechanic 1980:60). Thus, the family is seen as an ally and as a potentially constructive force in the care of their relative. Environmental practice accepts the family as a source for support, recognizing that the family is subject to considerable stress in coping with the disability of relatives (East 1992; Pilisuk and Parks 1988). Therefore, social support for the family itself is required to enhance their support for the service user (Auslander et al. 1993; Linsk et al. 1988; Cox, Parsons, and Kimboko 1988). Social support for the family is achieved through family support groups (Families Anonymous 1977).

Recognition of the importance of family support is evident in federal legislation in the areas of adult and child welfare. The Family Support Act of 1988 (Family Support Act 1988) provides for aid to persons on public welfare while the Family Support and Preservation Act of 1993 (Family Support and Preservation Act 1993) provides funds to enable children to remain with their natural families. Family preservation programs, which consist of intensive services in the home for the protection of children, have gained wide support, although their effectiveness has been questioned (Feldman 1991; Frankel 1988).

The importance of family support is being recognized through legislation in New Jersey that provides for welfare reform by an emphasis on services for the families of persons on public assistance (Family Development Act 1992). The Family Preservation Act of 1993 (Family Support and Preservation Act 1993) is similar to the federal legislation mentioned above in that it provides for services that enable children to remain with their natural families. A proposed law would produce a variety of support services to families of the developmentally disabled and chronically mentally ill. The Family Support Act of 1993 provides funding for service coordination, estate and transition planning, housing assistance, homemaker assistance, vocational and employment services, after school care, respite care, family education and training, medication education, self-advocacy training, and entitlement training (Family Support Act 1993). The Family Support Project taught informal supporters specific skills to help them cope with disabled relatives. Skills included modeling and role playing, behavioral rehearsal, coaching, social reinforcement; and performance feedback (Ferris and Marshall 1987). Another program provides family members with information and management skills (Iodice and Wodarsky 1987).

Utilization of support groups for caregivers to the frail elderly varies with factors linked to the amount of burden on the caregiver. Thus, those caring for Alzheimer's victims and elderly who had significant health problems had higher rates of attendance (Monahan et al. 1992).

Respite is another form of support for families in the day-to-day care of the disabled. Respite care services can include adult day care, home health care, and institutional care (Meltzer 1982). However, in-hospital respite as a moderator of caregiver stress can have negative consequences for Alzheimer's patients (Larkin and Hopcroft 1993).

Families also assume a role of indirect care provider–that of a case manager. In the absence of professional case management, families fill the void of service coordination. Especially in situations where relatives have a serious disability extending over a lengthy time period, some families develop specialized expertise on how to access community resources (Lowy 1985). Partnership between agencies and families can help facilitate the role of relatives as case managers (Seltzer, Ivry, and Lichfield 1992).

As indicated above, friends, neighbors, and significant others can provide somewhat different kinds of support to persons in need (Lechner 1993). These informal caregivers also require support if they are to function at their maximum capacity. Programs of professional consultation have been instituted for these informal caregivers to improve their helping functions (Froland et al. 1981:85). Caution needs to be taken that such professional consultation does not diminish these informal caregivers' natural instincts for helping and their tolerance of nonnormal functioning by introducing a sickness or problem emphasis.

Local merchants such as bartenders and hairdressers have been found to be important community caregivers (Cowen 1982). In general, the kinds of problems brought to them do not differ from those usually brought to mental health specialists (Gottlieb 1983:85). In the case situation, a family support group provided the daughter with relief of the stress associated with the conflict between her mother's support needs and her own personal needs.

Formal Caregivers

Support for formal caregivers is directed at such professional helpers as doctors, divorce lawyers, clergymen, social workers, and other employees of human-service organizations. Divorce lawyers, as compared to other community caregivers, are extensively involved with the psychosocial needs of their service consumers (Cowen 1982). Physicians in general practice are approached early in the help-seeking process, particularly in the case of "nervous conditions," psychosomatic disorders, and drug-related difficulties. In addition, they serve as gate keepers for public and private psychiatric services.

However, physicians tend not to be very responsive to patient's psychosocial problems (Harrison 1979). Given their key role as a source of community caregiving to patients in stress, it is important that efforts be made to provide them with the support they may require to handle the large number of patients with psychosocial problems who seek their aid.

The clergy are another important group of community caregivers who are approached by individuals undergoing transitional stresses (e.g., marriage, birth, death). Since churches today are moving more and more into the area of psychosocial counseling and support, they are prime candidates for support intervention programs. The New Jersey Division of Mental Health and Hospitals has funded a consulting service for churches, synagogues, and mental health centers to promote joint efforts to address the community-life needs of the long-term mentally ill (Holcomb 1985; Walters and Neugeboren 1995). In Connecticut, project ACCORD is an example of a collaborative aftercare program between a church and a mental health center (Anderson 1985).

Another form of social support to formal caregivers is that given to employees of human service agencies to minimize occupational stress and prevent burnout. Evidence indicates that the work environment of health organizations is less supportive than general work settings (Moos and Lemke 1983:156). Professionals employed in agencies serving critically ill and dying patients report more stress from the organizational environment than from work with patients (Vachon 1987 51-73). Job stress, especially during economic downturns, generates concerns about job entry, seniority, mobility, and pressures for job productivity. Considering the large amount of time spent on the job, stress associated with job overload, job ambiguity, reduced monetary compensation, poor prospects for job advancement, and the general strain of working in impersonal bureaucratic systems can result in occupational burnout in the human services (Neugeboren 1991:109-122).

Two kinds of support are possible: from supervisors and peers. Social support by supervisors has been found to have positive effects on job morale and productivity (Gottlieb 1983: 170-174). Six kinds of support can be made available from supervisors: listening, technical support, technical challenge, emotional support, emotional challenge, and feedback (Pines and Aronson 1981:29). Peer support in the workplace has been found to be less useful because of differences in values and theoretical orientations, status differences, and competition for scarce resources (Pines and Maslach 1978).

Community At Large

Targeting the community at large for intervention involves such activities as neighborhood helping; community empowerment; mutual-aid and event-centered programs; network-centered intervention; and linkage of informal and formal care systems. *Neighborhood helping* activities consist of assistance to key persons in the neighborhood who perform helping roles.

Community empowerment includes the organizing of informal leaders to promote the improvement of services. *Mutual-aid* groups are organized on behalf of a specific citizen group who are at risk because they are exposed to a common life crisis. The goal of *network-centered interventions* is to restructure people's networks in order to improve their helping processes and enlarge their access to social support (Gottlieb 1983:83).

Linking of formal and informal care systems involves strengthening informal helping activities. This is done by staff members expanding access to formal services by acting as bridges between formal and informal systems.

INTERVENTIONS

Intervention into social networks on behalf of the service user involves activities that pose some risk, since practitioner roles are ambiguous and public. Such interventions require a professional perspective that views the service consumer not only as an individual, but also as a part of a network.

Micro social-support interventions will now be discussed in terms of the organizational and community arenas of practice. Although arenas deal with direct service to individuals, a distinction is made regarding how the social network should be influenced. In the organizational arena of practice, the social network is a resource for service users or their families. Interventions are directed at influencing the network to assist the service consumer. In the community arena of practice, the social network itself becomes the target for intervention on behalf of groups of clients (see the conceptual model presented in Chapter 1). The professional role in the community arena is similar to the customary role of the community organizer in "locality development" (Rothman 1979).

Organizational Arena: Direct Practice

The discussion of intervention roles in the organizational arena of practice will first focus on preparatory interventions, then on network interventions, intervention in multiagency networks, intervention in family environments, and finally on different agency intervention strategies. This model of direct practice network interventions draws on the work of Gottlieb (1983).

Preparatory Interventions

In the direct-service process, the worker first engages in activities that are preparatory to the actual intervention into the personal network of the service user. This requires skills in assessment, screening, and anticipatory guidance.

Assessment. This process is directed at the individual's social, structural and interpersonal resources (Gottlieb 1983:108-115). It consists of an evaluation of the range of the service consumer's available support resources and how they can be used to improve the individual's situation. This assessment includes three separate appraisals of the primary social network: (1) determining its membership; (2) evaluating the balance of support vs. stress in the network; and (3) monitoring the network's response to professional intervention.

Determining the membership of the individual's primary social network involves first obtaining information on which persons inhabit current and past networks. This includes the nuclear and extended family, persons in the workplace, neighborhood and voluntary organizations (e.g., religious, civic, social), as well as other intimate role relations. The service user or other informants can provide this information, which is then used to determine how these networks connect with the person's current problem situation.

Evolving the balance of support vs. stress in the primary social network involves determining if social interactions are supportive or stressful. This assessment is based on the following types of supportive interactions: (1) emotional support; (2) cognitive guidance; (3) socializing and companionship; (4) environmental action; and (5) provision of material aid. The professional determines the support/stress balance by having the service consumer evaluate if support from a particular network member is helpful or not.

In *monitoring the lay system's responses to professional intervention,* the worker assesses the fit between service goals and the norms, expectations, and behavioral standards of network members. Lack of congruence can cause the service user to prematurely discontinue service. In order for service to be effective, it should be responsive to lay system beliefs and care.

In the case situation, the worker initially did an assessment of Mrs. S' support system, which included both the family and the neighborhood. She determined how Mrs. S felt about family and neighbors in terms of the support/stress involved in their relationships. The worker also showed sensitivity to the norms of the neighbors by presenting Mrs. S' problems as a natural outcome of the aging process.

Screening. Deciding whether the service user is suitable for referral to support groups requires screening to determine whether the individual has the ability to benefit from referral. The individual's social resources need to be evaluated, and if these are lacking, a determination must be made as to whether the deficiency in social contacts is due to lack of social skills, alienation, or simply a preference for coping alone (Schacter 1959). Decisions are required as to whether the individual needs help in order to be prepared for referral to a support group. The worker should also decide whether referral to a formal support group or access to informal sources of support is indicated. For example, it has been found that men resist referral to support groups. Gottlieb (1983:81) suggests that this resistance might be overcome if support groups were organized in the work situation.

In the case situation, the worker had to determine if Mrs. S was a suitable referral for a self-help group. This woman had not been a "joiner," and had so devoted her life to her family that her "social resources" were somewhat limited. Her lack of social contacts were related to her wish to cope without outside help. The worker therefore developed a plan to prepare her for referral that involved having her son, her doctor, and a person in a similar situation (a widow) talk to her about the value of going to a self-help group. The worker simultaneously expanded Mrs. S' access to informal sources of support by the contacts she made with the neighbors.

Anticipatory Guidance. This is used in situations where there is advance knowledge that a person will face life transitions. Such intervention can take the form of preretirement counseling; counseling for high school students entering college or full-time employment; premarital counseling; prenatal counseling, etc. In the case of Mrs. S, anticipatory guidance could have been done when her husband was terminally ill and it could be foreseen that his death would pose a traumatic life transition for this woman.

Assessment, screening, and anticipatory guidance procedures require the application of *decision-making skills.* Assessment relates to *problem definition*, in that a formulation is made of how a person's social network is linked with the particular problem being addressed. In the example, the worker evaluated the ways in which Mrs. S' relations with her family and neighbors were connected with her health problems and the solutions of these problems. The worker observed that Mrs. S had an independent nature and lacked social resources. In the screening procedure, the worker moved to the second stage of the decision-making process and conducted a *search for alternative solutions* to solve the problem. Such alternative solutions as referral to a self-help group and individual counseling were considered. Evaluation of the *costs vs. benefits* of these solutions took into account Mrs. S' natural reluctance to seek assistance and led to a plan that prepared her for referral to a self-help group. The worker discarded the alternative of individual counseling because of Mrs. S' reluctance to view her problem in psychological terms.

Network Interventions

There are several kinds of network interventions: network therapy (Speck and Atteneave 1973); social systems therapy (Pattison 1973); and the screening-linking-planning conference (Garrison 1974).

Network therapy is used when the service consumer has alienated his/her support system, and involves primary group members (close friends, family members, workmates) in therapeutic procedures. This type of intervention is fairly intensive, and requires about six hours of planning, implementation, and follow-up. It involves a certain amount of confrontation of conflict within the network. This type of intervention would have been appropriate in the case example because of the amount of alienation and conflict.

Social systems therapy is an extension of family therapy. Its focus is the "psychosocial kinship system," those people with whom the service user has frequent interaction, strong feelings of attachment, and mutual exchange of positive affect. It is used to mobilize resources during a crisis. This type of intervention was less appropriate for the case situation because of the absence of strong positive attachments in the kinship network.

The *screening-linking-planning conference* is practiced in crisis situations where the individual has been separated from his/her support system, as occurs during institutionalization. Its goal is to help ease transition to community life by restoring lost "environmental attachments." The goal of the intervention is to restore equilibrium by mobilizing feedback from persons in the intimate social network. This intervention method has been used to help drug offenders make the transition from inpatient to community settings (Callan, Garrison, and Zerger 1975).

These three network strategies have in common the objective of reestablishing mutually satisfying role relationships following a crisis. They are relevant for environmental practice because of the focus on the reweaving of social networks. These network approaches require the professional to view the service user as part of a network within which he/she has to achieve a balance between independence and dependence. In the example, the worker had the task of helping Mrs. S to reestablish an equilibrium between her increased dependency and her strong desire remain independent. The worker accomplished this by exerting influence on the social network of the family and neighborhood.

Intervention in Multiagency Networks

The focus of this kind of intervention is the network of agencies that impact on a service consumer. It is particularly relevant for low-income individuals who are served by several public and voluntary social service agencies. The target of intervention is not only of the service user, but also the agency providers, including the agreements that result from interagency coordination.

In the case situation, there was a problem of lack of coordination of medical services provided by physicians and pharmacists. The worker performed a coordinator role in having the doctors and the pharmacist work together with regard to the medications received by Mrs. S. This process necessitated the use of *negotiating* skills. The worker facilitated the cooperation between the doctor and druggist by showing them that it was in the self-interest of both parties to coordinate their efforts, since this was needed for the benefit of their patient, Mrs. S.

Intervention in Family Environments

A major intervention too used in family environments is the family support group. Family support groups can have educational, peer-support, and economic purposes. Educational support is obtained through the provision of information on the psychological, physical, and social aspects of a relative's disability including the expectations they can have of them. Psychoeducational programs with families of the mentally ill have reduced relapse rates (Falloon, Boyd, and McGill 1984). Peer support focuses on the caregiving roles in order to alleviate guilt associated with balancing personal needs and caregiver responsibilities. Economic support consists of direct financial assistance to the family, such as tax write-offs and direct money allotments to help cope with the financial expenses incurred in helping a disabled relative.

Different types of family environments can also have negative or positive consequences for relatives. "High expressed emotion" (e.g., criticism) (Brown, Birley, and Wing 1972; Vaughn and Leff 1976) by family members has deleterious effects on mentally ill relatives including high relapse rates, compared to families with low expressed emotion. In addition, spouses have higher expectations of returning mental patients than do parents, resulting in both higher functioning and higher relapse rates (Freeman and Simmons 1963).

These different family environments require interventions that takes these difficulties into account. Interventions to modify high levels of expressed emotion in the service consumer's home can be achieved by organizing support groups that combine high and low expressed-emotion families (Berkowitz et al. 1981). Similarly, support groups made up of a combination of conjugal and parental families would focus on how low and high expectations can have positive and negative effects. The three kinds of network interventions discussed above (network therapy, social systems therapy, and the screening-linking-planning conference) are also appropriate for intervening in family environments.

In the case situation, the daughter participated in a family support group. This group provided the daughter with educational as well as peer support. She learned to better understand her mother's difficulties through an appreciation of the problems of the bereaved elderly. Peer support helped her achieve a better balance between her responsibilities to her mother and her own personal needs.

Agency Intervention Strategies

Five different types of agency strategies have been formulated: personal networks; volunteer linking; mutual aid-self help; neighborhood helper; and community empowerment (Froland et al.

1981:64-65). These agency strategies utilize three types of staff/ helper relationships: coordinative, collegial, and directive. First we will address the five strategies, followed by a discussion of the types of staff/helper relationships.

Personal networks and volunteer linking are micro level organizational interventions and will be discussed here. Neighborhood helper and community empowerment will be discussed under micro level community interventions. Mutual aid self-help will be discussed in terms of both the organizational and community arenas of practice.

The *personal-network* strategy focuses on the person's individual network that provides assistance to reinforce the efforts of family, friends, and neighbors. Emphasis is on strengthening existing relationships, renewing old friendships, or establishing new ones. In this strategy, the staff/helper relationship is collegial. This strategy is used in service for the elderly, as was illustrated in the case.

Volunteer linking matches lay helpers to the service user to provide companionship, support, and advocacy. The purpose is to develop one-to-one relationships between people undergoing crisis and informal helpers who can provide the necessary support, advice, and personal commitment. This type of intervention is appropriate when existing sources of support are limited, and is useful for persons with long-term adjustment needs such as the developmentally disabled and the physically handicapped. Volunteers are recruited via advertising and other service consumers who have made successful adjustments. These volunteers can also serve as role models for the service user. A directive staff/helper relationship is used, involving training and supervision of the volunteer.

On the micro organizational level, the *mutual aid-self help strategy* consists of referral of those individuals who can benefit from mutual-aid and self-help groups. It will be recalled that the variation in structure of these two kinds of groups affect their appropriateness for persons who have different social capacities–mutual aid for those with more social resources and self-help for those with less. The case situation provides examples of the personal-network and self-help strategies. The social worker reinforced Mrs. S' personal network by strengthening her relationships with the family and neighbors. The self-help strategy was evident in the referral of Mrs. S to a group for widowed persons.

Volunteer linking, which involves recruitment of lay persons to connect them with service consumers, requires the use of *representing* skills to recruit volunteers. The staff person needs to represent the goals and procedures of this type of program in order to involve lay persons and former service users in this kind of program. *Leadership* skills are also required by the staff person who supervises the volunteer, and *staffing* skills are necessary in the training of the volunteer.

Types of Staff/Helper Relationships

Coordinative relations involve a relatively high degree of independent action. Collegial relations presuppose shared responsibility and authority. A directive relationship means that staff have the authority to supervise the informal helpers.

These three types of relationships have been associated with the different types of program intervention discussed above (Froland et al. 1981:66). The *personal-network strategy* is primarily *collegial,* while *volunteer linking* is *directive.* That aspect of *mutual aid-self help* involving the establishment of peer support groups is *collegial,* while that consisting of consulting with existing support groups is either *directive* or *coordinative. Neighborhood helpers* is a *collegial* strategy and *community empowerment* is *coordinative.* This formulation of staff/helper roles provides the micro environmental practitioner with a diversified approach for implementing the different types of agency-intervention strategies.

Having completed the discussion of interventions at the micro level of the orgranizational arena, we will now discuss interventions on the micro level of community practice.

Community Arena: Community Organization

The goal of community organization is to impact on local networks to enable them to function better. The community itself therefore becomes the target of intervention. The purpose of community organization is to help individuals who reside in the community achieve better integration with these networks.

The discussion of community interventions begins with a presentation of neighborhood assessment as an introduction to mutual aid–self-help, caregiver-centered support development, and community-empowerment network interventions.

Neighborhood Assessment

Since social networks vary in structure in different communities, it is important to determine the characteristics of the particular community in which the environmental practitioner works. At the neighborhood level, there are differences in the strength of ties, in the density of interconnections, and in the types of organizations within which ties are formed and maintained between neighborhoods. These variations among neighborhoods will affect the kinds of interventions used. Four criteria serve as a framework for doing a neighborhood assessment: community homogeneity; cultural traditions; population stability; and integrating institutions (Froland et al. 1981:140-146).

Community homogeneity is a measure of community diversity in terms of race, ethnicity, social status, life-cycle stage, and kinship. Differences in race, ethnicity, and class can act as barriers to informal helping exchanges. In an elderly white community where young African-Americans moved in, age and race differences were a barrier to developing informal helping (Froland et al. 1981:141).

Cultural traditions generate norms and values that can help or hinder the informal helping process. For example, norms of self-reliance can be a barrier to mutual aid. Similarly, a strong family-based culture will hinder helping activities. Practitioners with few preconceptions are likely to encounter less resistance than those who have a set model that is not responsive to the particular community's cultural needs.

Population stability provides a base of relationships upon which social networks can be built. Transient communities, or ones in transition, pose barriers for the development of informal helping. Interventions will have to be modified to adapt to such characteristics. For example, population a volunteer consisting of college students will require a rotating system.

Integrating institutions are behavior settings that facilitate interaction among people (Barker et al. 1978). An example of a behavior setting would be a grocery store that has a snack bar where people can linger. Institutions like schools, churches, libraries, cafes, and businesses that serve a local area can be influential in uniting people within a neighborhood. The micro community practitioner needs to become aware of these behavior settings to be able to use them for support for the service consumer.

In the case situation, the social worker determined that Mrs. S lived in a homogeneous and stable community whose cultural traditions inhibited close personal friendships outside the family. She used a "behavior setting" of tenants who congregated in front of the building.

This neighborhood assessment procedure required the worker to use *decision-making* skills. First, the specific neighborhood had to be assessed in relation to Mrs. S' problem. Understanding of the barriers to informal helping imbedded in the norms of the community helped in the search for solutions to Mrs. S' problem. Then the cost vs. the benefits of different solutions to Mrs. S' problem had to be evaluated given the context of the particular community in which she lived.

Community Interventions

Community interventions that will be discussed include: (1) Self-help and event-centered networks; (2) caregiver-centered support development activities; (3) community-empowerment network interventions; and (4) linkage of formal and informal care systems. It must be kept in mind that intervention by community organizers uses the individual needs of groups of clients as the basis for intervening in the community system.

Self-Help and Event-Centered Networks. Community organizers develop self-help and event-centered support groups for those persons who are exposed to a common life crisis. Support is appropriate for such event-centered life crises as bereavement, marital separation, retirement, unemployment, job and school transition, geographic relocation; and since these events have a destabilizing impact. A secondary purpose of event-centered support groups is the assimilation of group members in one another's ongoing social networks to increase mutual-aid activities in people's lives.

Micro community intervention in self-help networks involve community organizers in the following activities: consulting to support existing networks; creating mutual-aid networks; and organizing mutual-aid groups for advocacy purposes.

Consultation to support existing networks establishes ties to the service user's existing self-help groups to provide assistance to maintain their functioning. *Creating new self-help networks* involves contacting present and former service consumers and informal caregivers to establish new self-help groups. Professionally initiated support groups provide support for the bereaved (Silverman et al. 1974); those making the transition to parenthood (McGuire and Gottlieb 1979); and parents of premature infants (Minde et al. 1980). Silverman (1980) developed a manual for use by professionals for the organization of self-help groups. It includes methods for defining and locating populations in need, creating the organization, designing initial meetings, selecting mutual-help activities, and overcoming problems that develop within groups.

Organizing mutual-aid groups for advocacy purposes occurs particularly among parents of the disabled. Parents of the mentally retarded have developed an effective nationwide advocacy organization (Alliance for the Mentally Ill). Parents of the mentally ill organized to pressure for legislative changes that protect their childrens' rights.

In the case example, the community organizer helped to create a new self-help group, Medical Alert. This group successfully advocated for financial support for medical alarms for the disabled elderly in the community.

Intrinsic to creating new self-help groups are the skills of *representing* and *leadership. Representing* is needed to enlist support from funding authorities to obtain the resources needed to establish new organizations. *Leadership* is necessary to influence persons in positions of authority to support the creation of new agencies. These skills are also appropriate for advocacy activities.

Caregiver-Centered Support Development Activities. The primary aim of network-centered interventions is to strengthen the capacity of social networks to provide ongoing and crisis support in advance of any stressors. The purpose is to facilitate informal caregiving roles and processes. These interventions can be directed at informal caregivers and/or existing social networks. They are used for settings where people tend to be socially isolated or marginal, and where social networks are resource deficient or structurally too weak to provide adequate support.

Intervention by community organizers with informal caregivers emphasizes equality in status. The professional must be careful not to assume a supervisory role. Information is provided to facilitate referral to self-help groups.

Interventions to support formal caregivers focus on educating the caregiver about the ways in which the service user's tendency to comply with professional directives, such as the suggestions of doctors and lawyers, will be influenced by their social network. Intervention programs have been conducted with such caregivers as divorce attorneys and hairdressers (Doane 1977; Weisenfeld and Weiss 1979).

Interventions in neighborhood helping networks, focus on assisting key figures in the neighborhood who are performing informal helping roles. This activity recognizes that neighborhood helpers can strengthen mutual-aid among residents and help integrate isolated persons into the community. The first task of the community organizer is to identify these neighborhood helpers. This is done by talking with community residents to determine which have reputations as helpers. The professional enlists the aid of these informal helpers to integrate socially isolated persons into community activities. The professional can provide concrete resources (e.g., transportation to community activities) to enable the service user and the neighborhood helper to establish linkages.

In the case situation, the worker discovered that one of the tenants of the apartment house was active in helping others. The professional encouraged this person to take responsibility for enlarging the medical alarm program and thereby increased mutual helping among the tenants.

Influencing formal caregivers and neighborhood helpers requires *leadership* skills. This involves the ability to use referent and expert power to persuade these parties to participate in cooperative efforts to enhance social networks.

Community-Empowerment Network Interventions. The community organizer empowers the community by organizing informal leaders to promote the improvement of existing services and the development of new programs. In contrast to neighborhood helping, community empowerment has a political emphasis. It mobilizes community leaders with ties to the informal helping network to represent the interests of the service users. The community organizer plays a coordinative role in facilitating meetings and helping focus on issues leading to community problem solving. An important goal of this type of intervention is community ownership of the newly developed programs. Since community empowerment is a political process, different community interests will be in competition. The professional has to be aware of the likely dominance of provider interests in order to balance them with service consumers' interests.

In the case situation, the community organizer mobilized community leaders to address the problem of the lack of coordination in the prescribing and dispensing of drugs to the elderly. Her efforts resulted in the empowerment of the local community through the creation of a community organization that could devise solutions to problems common to the elderly, such as drug overmedication.

Community-empowerment interventions involve community organizing activities that necessitate *leadership* and *negotiating* skills. Mobilizing community leaders requires the ability to use expert and referent power to influence key persons in the community to act jointly. Negotiating skills are required to persuade different interest groups to join together even if it means compromising their interests.

Linking of Formal and Informal Care Systems. The purpose of linking formal and informal care systems is to enhance informal helping by increasing access to formal services. Successful linkage with the informal system has to take into account the informal-care norms of mutual-aid, self-determination, and self-reliance. In the case, a linkage was established between the family service agency and the informal neighborhood support networks.

Linkage of formal and informal care systems uses *negotiating* skills. The self-interests of the formal and informal systems are merged on the basis that an exchange of resources will be to the benefit of both systems.

SUMMARY

This chapter on micro level social support first discussed several issues surrounding social support intervention including cost vs.

benefits, integration of formal and informal care, and the potential for preventive interventions. A definition of social support was presented which encompassed the roles of both formal and informal care systems. Formal care interventions were viewed as bolstering and facilitating the work of informal care systems. Social support included mutual-aid, self-help, and community-support systems. Targets of social support included service users, informal and formal caregivers, and the community at large.

Social support interventions on the micro level were discussed in terms of the organizational and community arenas of practice. In the organizational arena, topic areas covered included preparatory, family, informal network, agency, and multiagency interventions. In the community arena, the topics discussed were neighborhood assessment and community interventions.

Throughout this chapter, the principles and intervention strategies were illustrated through application to a case situation presented at the beginning of the chapter. A discussion of the intervention skills in Chapter 2 was integrated with the explication of social support interventions.

STUDY QUESTIONS

1. You are a direct-service practitioner in a program for the chronically mentally ill. A service consumer assigned to you is being discharged from an in-patient facility. What discharge plans would you make for support of this person in the community? What kinds of practice skills would you need to accomplish this task?

2. An elderly disabled service user has been assigned to you. She has no family or close friends, but had been active in her local church. What actions would you take to develop social support for this person to help avoid placement in a nursing home? What practice skills would you use?

3. An adolescent in your caseload suffers from drug and alcohol addiction. The parents are very worried and are developing various health problems as a result of the stress they are under. What case plan using social support would you make to deal with this situation?

4. The wife of an intravenous drug abuser who recently was diagnosed with AIDS comes to you, a community organizer, for assistance. She informs you that there are other women in her neighborhood who are in a similar situation. She has tried to help these other women, but she is overwhelmed because of the lack of services for persons with AIDS. What steps would you take to help this woman to organize support services in the community to deal with the problem of AIDS? Indicate the kind of practice skills you would need to accomplish the task of "empowering" this community group.

5. Review the case presented at the beginning of this chapter and discuss whether the social worker was intrusive in her efforts to intervene in this situation.

6. You are a marital counselor and have become aware that many persons contemplating divorce have had stress-related problems that their lawyers do not understand. These problems often result in complications in the divorce proceedings, prolonging the process and compounding the psychological and economic difficulties. What kind of program would you develop with the service consumers and attorneys to deal with this problem?

7. You work in an employee assistance program and have become aware of employees developing health problems shortly after retirement. Develop a plan for social support services to deal with this situation.

8. You have a new person assigned to you for help. You need to do an assessment of this individual's social network. Discuss how you would go about doing a social network assessment. Indicate the kind of practice skills needed to do this assessment.

9. You are a community organizer and have been assigned the task of doing a neighborhood assessment. What criteria would you use for this assessment and how would go about completing this task?

10. Your task is to determine if there are any individuals in the neighborhood where you are working who are assuming helping roles. How would you find out who these people are? Having determined who they are, how would you facilitate their efforts?

Chapter 7

SOCIAL SUPPORT
ON THE MACRO LEVEL

Social Support
on the Macro Level

INTRODUCTION

Social support on the macro level involves the activities of the direct-service agency administrator, the community planner, and the policy analyst in developing and implementing social support policies and programs. Administrators of such direct-service agencies as mental health centers serving the severely mentally ill, social services agencies responsible for programs for the disabled elderly, health-care programs for the physically handicapped, and after care programs for the developmentally disabled should formulate agency social support goals and design and supervise organizational structures to implement them.

Community planners have similar objectives on the community level. Community needs assessments are done to determine the programs required for more supportive neighborhood environments. Creating such an environment can be facilitated by the integration of physical with social planning. For example, the social impact of such projected community changes as highway construction and urban renewal would need to be evaluated to prevent dysfunctional consequences to community supports. Community planners also can enhance informal community social networks as a means of fostering increased social support in the community.

Finally, social policy analysts working in legislative and administrative policy-formulating agencies can impact on the policy and procedures for the design and funding of social support programs.

This chapter begins with a presentation of a case situation that will be utilized for our discussion of social support on the macro level, followed by an examination of issues related to this topic area. Macro level interventions in the organizational, community, and societal arenas are then discussed, along with an examination of how the practice skills discussed in Chapter 2 relate to these macro intervention roles. Finally, the integration of micro and macro social support are addressed. It will be useful for the reader to be familiar with the *definitions* of social support discussed in Chapter 5 before reading this chapter.

CASE: CENTRAL COUNTY
SERVICES FOR THE AGED

The aged in Central County receive comprehensive social services from the Central County Association for Aging (CCAA). Social services planning for this population group is the responsibility of the Central County United Way and the State Department of Health and Welfare.

Ms. Mary Wilson was recently hired to direct the CCAA, which offers an array of programs including health care, meals on wheels, day care, family counseling, R.S.V.P., and homemaker services. A prime purpose of the CCAA is to enable the frail elderly to live in the community and avoid placement in nursing homes. It has a staff of social workers, nurses, case aides, and homemakers. The agency has several departments, including social service, nursing, home care, and day care. It is a nonprofit organization under a board of directors and is funded by the United Way and state grants.

Agency Goals

The former director was recently replaced by Ms. Wilson because of the funding authorities' dissatisfaction with the accomplishments of the programs under the agency's jurisdiction. These programs were not able to help service users who did not need protective care to continue to live in the community. The new administrator's initial assessment determined that the goal of maintaining the frail elderly in the community was not being accomplished because the social service staff was not giving adequate attention to the provision of social support services. Further examination of the official policies revealed that they were somewhat ambiguous as to whether emphasis should be on people-changing therapeutic services or environmental social support.

Plan for Changing the Agency

Ms. Wilson developed a plan, with the board's approval, for changing the goals and structures of this agency. The director formulated a new statement of agency goals that stressed the provision of social support services. She obtained the board's support by presenting data on the effectiveness of social support interventions in community programs for the disabled elderly. She established a new social support department that had the authority to coordinate all of the agency's services. This was done because it was evident that there was inadequate cooperation between the different organizational units resulting in the lack of coordination of services for the service consumers. Staff recruitment stressed the community skills needed to work with formal and informal helping networks. Educational techniques were also emphasized, since staff were expected to give information to service users and their families on the technical aspects of their problems. Since lack of adequate housing was a significant problem, the director created another new unit within the social support department that was responsible for locating housing for service users.

The administrator next evaluated the personnel policies regarding promotion and merit raises. These were modified, with successful performance measured in terms of positive functioning of the elderly in the community. Finally, Ms. Wilson established a resource coordination unit within the new social support department that had the responsibility for interagency coordination, including the development of affiliation agreements. One such agreement was made with the local public housing authority.

Overcoming the Resistance to Change

The director met with staff and informed them of the funding authority's dissatisfaction with the program's accomplishments. She informed them of her plans for changing the goals and structure of the agency. The responses were somewhat negative, especially those of the social workers. They were convinced that family counseling was the service most needed by the service consumers. They were unwilling to learn new social support techniques.

Ms. Wilson developed a plan for implementating of the change from a therapeutically oriented program to one that stressed social support. She started by hiring new supervisory staff with experience in social support programs. These supervisors worked with the administrator in developing job descriptions for the staff that specified social support roles and functions. These new job expectations were communicated to the staff. It was explained that their work would be evaluated in terms of the specific standards established in these job specifications. As a result of these new expectations, a number resigned and obtained employment in other agencies.

The staff vacancies provided the administrator with the opportunity to recruit new staff with interest and skills in social support interventions. She developed an instrument that simulated social support interventions for use in the hiring process. She could, therefore, screen applicants, and select those who best qualified to fill the positions available. Ms. Wilson also recruited a supervisor for staff development who developed a program to train both old and new staff in social support intervention techniques. Line supervisors were also trained to provide the technical support to their staff that helped them deal with job pressures, with the result that staff morale was enhanced. An evaluation and monitoring system was linked to the new job expectations and integrated with the agency's promotion and merit-pay procedures. Program-evaluation staff developed a reporting system that provided data on staff activities and service user outcomes, including whether they were being placed in nursing homes.

Community Needs

A variety of social support programs were introduced, including: (1) mutual-aid and self-help groups for service users, their families, and informal and formal caregivers; and (2) consultation to neighborhood social networks. Although these interventions were helpful for the service users, the staff reported to the administrator that there were certain neighborhoods where social networks were fragmented or underdeveloped. In one low-income neighborhood, plans for redevelopment were threatening to disrupt the existing social networks of a number of elderly.

This information on community needs was communicated by the administrator to the United Way, which was the agency responsible for social planning to enhance the quality of life in the community. This agency had created network-development workshops that focused on enhancing the informal aspects of community life.

The community social planner, upon learning about the potential adverse effects of redevelopment on the social support systems of low-income elderly, contacted the county planning board, which was considering a real estate development plan to build an office building and condominiums. With the aid of members of his board and a local state assemblyman, the community planner petitioned the county planning board to include an evaluation of the social impact of the redevelopment as part of their environmental impact assessment. The planning board asked the United Way to do this social assessment. Their report resulted in a modification of the redevelopment plans to include low-income housing for the elderly.

New Legislation

The Central County United Way funded a variety of programs for severely disabled persons, including the frail elderly. This agency became aware that the state Rehabilitation Act, passed ten years earlier, was not achieving its purpose of helping the disabled remain in the community. The United Way presented information documenting this to the state legislator who originally sponsored the statute. He turned the matter over to his policy analyst.

The legislative aide reviewed the statute and determined that the law had the goal of maintaining the handicapped in the community by two means: rehabilitation and social support. The social support objective was to be achieved through programs of coordination of formal and informal systems of care.

The aide obtained information on the implementation of the programs funded under the Rehabilitation Act from the State Department of Health and Welfare. The information dealt with the kinds of programs being conducted and data on the impact of these programs on the disabled. For the most part, the agencies serving the handicapped justified their programs on the basis of effort rather than results. The aide also learned that many of the disabled were being inappropriately institutionalized, and that the primary thrust of the program was on rehabilitation rather than social support. In addition, minimal effort had been made to coordinate services for the severely disabled. He also determined that while an interweaving of formal and informal care was mandated in the law, in practice, formal care was not provided when informal care was available.

The policy analyst also reviewed the research literature on social support and discovered that there was much potential for preventive programs. He determined that other states had established programs to improve the quality of community life. Specifically, community physical redevelopment statutes now required a social impact analysis to obtain approval of new highway and commercial construction.

The aide recommended the following modifications of the Rehabilitation Act to the state assemblyman, who incorporated them in a new bill:

1. Specify that the goal of the law was to avoid institutional placement by the use of social support intervention programming.
2. Establish specific criteria for the objective of coordinating formal and informal care programs.
3. Add a provision for prevention programs focused on improving community support systems.
4. Add a provision specifying that evaluation of the extent that service users were able to be maintained in the community will be performed.
5. Establish mechanisms for interagency coordination.

ISSUES

There are several issues that pertain to macro practice in the social support area. These relate to the general problem of giving priority to environmentally oriented social support interventions, rather than to the traditional people-changing service modalities. Three interrelated issues are relevant to this major policy shift: (1) consensus vs. power strategies (Neugeboren 1991:203-205) for achieving a social support program shift; (2) creation of new agencies vs. the use of existing human-service programs to accommodate social support objectives; and (3) the role of the lay community in accomplishing this policy change.

Consensus vs. Power Strategies for Achieving Social Support for Program Changes

What change strategy is required to accomplish a shift to social support programming? Should one look to a consensus strategy, relying on persuasion as the main approach for convincing adminis-trators and line practitioners to adopt the new social support-inter-ventions approaches to service? Will professionals and lay persons who control agency boards be able to modify their ideological convictions that people-changing interventions are the most ap-propriate ones? Will line staff who have invested many years in traditional service technologies be inclined to give up these tech-niques and take the time and effort to learn the new social support approaches (Whittaker et al. 1983:59). Since this policy change will of necessity involve a redistribution of power and control over programs from those who support traditional people-changing in-tervention to those advocating social support, can this be achieved on a voluntary basis?

If persuasion is not a viable strategy, should power be used to impose the change? Should administrators, planners, and policy analysts mandate the change, establish procedures for recruiting staff who will support social support programming, and sanction staff who are not willing or able to provide this kind of program-ming? Given the existing power structure in the human services field, is it politically feasible to introduce such a mandated change?

If neither a consensus nor a power strategy is feasible, then what is the potential for forgoing efforts to change the existing human service agencies and creating new agencies specifically designed for social support intervention programming. This is a second issue worthy of discussion.

Creation of New Social Support Agencies

The strategy of bypassing existing human service agencies and creating new organizations was used in the poverty programs in the 1960s (Marris and Rein 1973). This strategy was based on the assumption that since existing welfare institutions were not able to address the needs of the poor, new agencies were needed to accom-plish this purpose. The power and resources to do this first came from the Ford Foundation and then, under the Kennedy and John-son administrations, from the federal government. National public policy provided the impetus for substantial funding for these new agency structures.

In the 1980s, public social policy has moved from the national to state and local levels. Under the Reagan administration, federal funding for social programming has been reduced, with the states filling in some of the gaps. Given this environment, would it be politically feasible for the states to embark on a program of creating new agencies to achieve social support program goals? Are the demographic changes of an aging society and the concomitant increase in the political influence of senior citizens a possible foundation for support for the creation of a new human service system that is based on social support? We see evidence of new social support organizations being created to fill the vacuum resulting from the unwillingness or inability of traditional agencies to serve the severely mentally ill. The increased visibility of the homeless is placing pressure on authorities to examine policies and programs for the disabled, including housing policies. Direct-service agency administrators, community planners, and policy analysts may be in a position to use this changing environment that makes it politically feasible to create new programs for social support.

Role of Lay Community in Achieving Programming Change

In Chapter 6, we discussed "community empowerment" as an objective for social support intervention. The strategy of using the local citizenry in the promotion of social change was employed in the social action programs of the 1960s. What is the current potential for organizing local communities to foster the achievement of a change to social support programming?

There are signs that local communities can and will organize to deal with social problems confronting them. In response to such problems as crime, drug addiction, and homelessness, communities are organizing on the local level. For example, churches have sponsored housing for the homeless. These efforts appear to be taking place without much professional involvement. Is there a climate today for greater leadership of local citizenry in the organization of new social support programs (Clark 1988)? As indicated in Chapter 6, local citizens are a critical aspect of social networks.

Now that the issues related to social support on the macro level has been discussed, we will consider different macro level interventions in the organizational, community, and societal arenas.

INTERVENTIONS

Organizational Arena: Direct-Service Agency Administrator

The direct-service agency administrator provides the leadership needed for the agency to achieve social support service-delivery goals. Drawing on the model presented in Chapter 1, the management tasks involved are (1) formulating agency goals; (2) designing appropriate organizational structures; and (3) directing staff in the implementation of these goals.

Formulation of Goals of Social Support

Formulation of organizational social support goals requires the administrator to gain sanction from funding authorities, governing boards, and staff to give priority to social support goals. The establishment of official goals of social support is necessary in order to legitimate the allocation of resources to this programming function. The formulation of official goals also provides the mandate required to successfully shift agency priorities and to overcome resistance from those who have commitments to the more traditional modalities (Neugeboren 1991:182-188).

The case situation presented at the beginning of the chapter illustrates the role of the administrator in formulating organizational goals. This was a necessary first step in redirecting the agency toward social support programming. Formulation of organizational goals required the administrator to use *decision-making* and *representing* skills.

The decision-making skill involved *analyzing the problem* of the agency's failure to achieve the goal of maintaining the disabled elderly in the community. This analysis determined that the official goals were ambiguous with regard to therapeutic vs. social support modalities. In the *search for alternative solutions* to the problem, the administrator considered the possibility of prevention, counseling, and social support interventions. After the *evaluation of the costs and benefits* of different alternative solutions, the decision was made to use social support as the prime means for achieving the goal of maintaining these disabled service consumers in the community.

Representing skills were used to "sell" board and funding authorities on the need to formulate new organizational goals. The administrator had to present information on the lack of achievement of agency goals. To further convince the board, she used data to show that social support interventions were effective in programs for the disabled elderly.

Design of Organizational Structures

The successful achievement of social support goals depends on having the kinds of structures that will facilitate the accomplishment of these objectives in place. This requires the design of role, communication, reward, authority, and interorganizational structures (Neugeboren 1991:60)

The *role* structure specifies job definitions and descriptions. These job definitions apply to both direct-service and supervisory positions. As indicated previously, professional activities in the area of social support are different from those in practice directed at people-changing objectives. Knowledge of and skill in work with groups, organizations, and communities needs to be incorporated in position descriptions (Pancoast, Parker, and Froland 1983:48). Advance specification of the role structure required to achieve social support goals leads to procedures for recruitment, hiring, training, deployment, and monitoring of staff to assure that these goals will be carried out.

In the case situation, the administrator designed new job descriptions for the social service staff that incorporated community and educational tasks that were essential for social support interventions. Design of organizational roles required *staffing* skills to set guidelines for staff recruitment, selection, training, and performance evaluations. A clear definition of job responsibilities was essential in advertising for appropriate staff. In the hiring process, precise role definitions were needed in the design of the selection instrument. Training of old and new staff was also dependent on a clear understanding of job expectations. Finally, the development of a staff-appraisal system required the specification of performance roles.

Design of *communication structures* (i.e., who communicates with whom) is necessary to assure that different staff coordinate their efforts in accomplishing social support goals. Discharge-planning activities require specific communication between service providers within and outside the agency to insure that the service user is able to maintain support relationships. In the case, the problem of lack of communication between the different departments was dealt with by the establishment of a new social support department that was given the responsibility for interdepartmental coordination.

Design of communication structures to achieve coordination involves the *negotiating* skill. The administrator used this skill to facilitate the integration of the different departments in the agency by having the staff become aware of their interdependencies based on shared goals of service user benefit as well as the opportunity to exchange resources.

Changes in the *authority structure* are necessary to insure that social support activities have the sanction of persons in positions of authority. As indicated previously, sanction for the innovation of any new program is critical to overcoming organizational resistance to change. The organizational unit that is given responsibility for social support programming would need to be on a high enough level in the organization to have the authority and power to carry out its function. The newly created Department of Social Support was given the responsibility and authority of coordinating the different subunits to work toward the organization's goal of maintaining the disabled elderly in the community.

In contrast to the centralized structure suggested above for the *initiation* of program, a decentralized structure is recommended for the *operation* of programs (Froland et al. 1981:168). This facilitates the flexibility of "front line" staff in working with informal care systems. The decentralization of organizational structures has also been found to facilitate community placement of the disabled elderly (Prager and Shnit 1985).

Design of the authority structure is illustrated in the case as the new social support department was given the authority to coordinate the agency's support services. This aspect of organizational design facilitated the administrator's use of *leadership* skill. Ms. Wilson's ability to gain the cooperation of staff was enhanced by creating a structure that reinforced the agency's influencing staff to work toward social support goals.

The design of the *reward structure* is important to assure that social support objectives are achieved. Rewards for successful implementation of social support programs should be specified in advance to help motivate staff to work toward this goal. This is illustrated in the case by the revision of the personnel policies to link staff promotion and merit raises to the successful community adjustment of service consumers. The redesign of the reward structure also facilitated Ms. Wilson's *leadership* responsibilities, as it helped motivate staff to work for the agency's objectives.

Since social support programming requires collaboration between different human service agencies, the administrator should plan the *interorganizational structure.* Lack of effective interorganizational relations is a major barrier to interweaving formal and informal care systems (Pancoast, Parker, and Froland 1983:48). Fundamental to the promotion of more-structured relations between agencies is the promulgation of interagency contracts and agreements.

In the case, the director created a new resource coordination unit to develop procedures to link this agency's services with others in the community. This new structure facilitated the administrator's ability to use *negotiation* skills. This occurred when the resource unit provided information that the goals of the public housing agency were congruent with those of the CCAA. This led to the negotiation of an agreement for housing for their service users.

Program Implementation

A important objective of *program implementation* is the maintenance of social support for the service user during their involvement with the agency. For example, in such institutional settings as hospitals for persons with acute and chronic disease, action must be taken to prevent the service user from being disconnected from community supports. Different organizational arrangements are required for short-term acute-care patients than for persons in long-term chronic care.

In acute-care hospitals, policies should provide for relatives and friends to be with patients during critical stages of service. Similarly, discharge-planning functions should take place at the time of admission. Discharge planning has to take into account the role that informal supportive networks can play in the discharge.

For long-term patients, there is a greater risk that the service user will be disconnected from social supports in the community (Wells and Singer 1985:320). This is especially the case for persons whose disabilities have placed great burdens on informal caregivers. Support groups for family members will minimize disconnection of the service user from such support. Therefore, the administrative staff should develop family support programs. Persons with such long-term disabilities as mental illness and retardation are institutionalized for lengthy periods not because of their need for protective care, but due to a lack of supportive care in the community. It is the responsibility of the administrator of nursing homes, mental hospitals, and similar facilities to develop programs that will provide this aftercare. As in short-term institutions, discharge planning in long-term care facilities should start at the time of admission. This has implications for the role and skills of admission staff, which in turn affects recruitment and training procedures.

Organizational policies that encourage self-sufficiency and self-direction among residents of institutions will result in better social integration into the community (David, Moos, and Kahn 1981). Positive staff attitudes toward family during visits is associated with increased contact of institutionalized elderly residents with the outside world (Tobin and Kulys 1981). These findings suggest tasks for the administrator in the recruitment and training of staff that are oriented to facilitating community integration of residents through links with informal supports in the community (Wells and Singer 1985:320).

The case illustrates how the administrator facilitated the accomplishment of social support objectives through the performance of various administrative tasks. Recruitment and hiring of staff who had the skill to do this kind of work was a first step in moving the agency toward social support goals. Creating the position of supervisor for staff development met the need for training of old and new staff in social support technologies. A new monitoring and staff evaluation system linked to social support goals served to reinforce the accomplishment of these goals.

The evaluation of agency programs required the administrative staff to be proficient in *monitoring* skills. Verifying whether the agency is accomplishing social support objectives to achieve the goal of maintaining service consumers in the community requires that program evaluation staff have skill in obtaining data on staff activities and the results of these activities. The tasks involved in monitoring included development of a reporting system whereby staff provided information on their activities and outcome data on service users. Verifying the accomplishment of agency goals requires skill in obtaining data from staff and using spot checks to determine if the information is accurate.

As indicated in Chapter 6, social support for staff of human-service agencies can help minimize occupational burnout. This type of support can also have positive consequences for those being served. Poor morale of staff can have deleterious effects on residents (Stanton and Schwartz 1954). The administrator therefore has the responsibility of developing personnel policies and organizational structures that provide for staff support.

The Work Environment Scale (WES) (Moos 1981) is an evaluative tool that can be used by administrators to diagnose and change dysfunctional agency environments. It contains three dimensions: (1) relationships (involvement, peer cohesion, and supervisory support); (2) personal growth and goal orientation (autonomy, task orientation, and work pressure); and (3) system maintenance and change (clarity, control, innovation, and physical comfort). Data derived from the use of WES was used to decrease depression among women workers (Wetzel 1978) and to ameliorate stress in hospitals (Moos and Lemke 1983:157-158). This instrument was used to systematically assess and intervene to change dysfunctional organizational environments by feedback to staff of the negative aspects of their work settings (Moos 1979a, 1979b).

In the case situation, the provision of technical support by line supervisors enhanced staff morale by helping staff deal with the technical demands of the job. This supervisory role required *leadership* skills, which included the provision of technical supportive supervision (Austin 1981:300). This provided social support for the subordinates, enhancing their morale and reducing the possibility of burnout.

Intrinsic to policies and programs for insuring continuing social support of service users and informal caregivers is the dissemination of information to them as to the nature of the disability (Walsh 1988).

This includes the kinds of limitations present, and, perhaps more important, the areas of potential strength (Maluccio 1981; Rothman 1994:8). Provision of information to service users about their illness facilitates compliance with medical regimes for heart patients, such as smoking less and altering diets (Hackett 1978). Therefore, an important program that administrators can establish is that of education with informal caregivers (Black, Dornan, and Allegrante 1986). This educationally focused intervention has implications for skills required by staff, which in turn affects recruitment, training, supervision, and monitoring of staff. The case illustrates the importance of recruitment of staff with educational skills. Instructional competency is intrinsic to the training role included under the *staffing* skill.

We have discussed the role of the direct-service agency administrator in relation to social support programs. Next, we present the role of the community planner.

Community Arena: Community Planner

The goal of intervention by community planners in the area of social support is to extend and fortify the support aspects of community life. Deficiencies in community social support are determined through a needs assessment. The gaps in community support are rectified by promoting of social support programming through the provision of incentives to agencies to establish such programs. A more direct approach is the sponsorship of network-centered support-development workshops. A third approach is the facilitating of supportive agency environments.

Promotion of Social Support Programs

Community planners promote new program development by exerting different kinds of influence on the provider agencies they fund. Criteria for funding allocations should give priority to social support programs. Informal community leaders and representatives from self-help and mutual-aid groups should be included on committees responsible for allocation of program funds as a counter-balance to the traditional agency providers. In line with a planning agency's function of *facilitating interagency coordination,* grants for program development in the social support area should require affiliation agreements between interdependent support programs as a precondition for funding. This reduces the possibility of duplication of agency services. For example, a child protection agency and a school serving the same service consumer could develop agreements as to who will have the responsibility for developing social support programs. Nonfinancial incentives such as guarantee of publicity (Pancoast, Parker, and Froland 1983:44) should also be offered.

Network Development Workshops

A more direct approach that community planning agencies can take to enhance community social support is the sponsorship of a network-development workshop. This program has a primary prevention purpose in its restructuring of social networks to improve their helping processes and to enlarge their access to social support. It is aimed at altering those aspects of the community environment that create stress. Public education is the general strategy that is used to influence the community residents to be aware of and reduce environmental hazards. Network-development activities are based on research on how help-seeking behavior and primary group relations underlie quality of life (Campbell 1981). Network development workshops have three purposes: (1) help citizens improve their personal social networks (Todd 1980); (2) strengthen network helping processes (D'Augelli et al. 1981); and (3) preserve existing support networks (Gottlieb 1985:296-298).

Helping community residents to *improve their personal social networks* can lead to their planning ways to develop an integrated and supportive network. Understanding that diversity in social supports is functional and that there is an interplay between personal and social resources can help them optimize their access to social resources.

Strengthening network helping processes helps informal caregivers improve their caring skills. The goal of this training is to help the informal caregiver to positively change the nature of the informal caregiving system.

The case illustrates how a community planning agency can develop a program for improving the informal caregiving aspects of the community. Influencing informal care networks required the community planner to use *leadership* skills based on the expertise of the norms of informal care. The planner selectively introduced support to enhance the natural functioning of these networks. Training, which is part of the *staffing* skill, was also used to enable informal care leaders to function better in their roles.

Preserving existing support networks focuses on the negative effects of physical changes on the community (e.g., the disruption to neighborhood support systems caused by urban redevelopment). (Fried 1963). Since stability of residence in neighborhoods fosters social support, efforts to counteract the displacement of residents are crucial. For example, such financial arrangements as "equity sharing" allow residents to purchase their apartments and thereby prevent eviction because of conversion of their apartments to condominiums. Another housing support program is "shared housing," in which residents obtain help to set up joint living arrangements (Gottlieb 1983:100). The integration of social and physical planning (Morris and Frieden 1968) provides an opportunity for community social planners to link up with community physical planning boards to insure that the social consequences of physical changes are taken into account. Environmental impact studies, which are required when major construction is planned (e.g., highways), should also include an evaluation of the social impact.

The case illustrates how a social planner can diminish the negative effects of real estate redevelopment on community life by contributing "social impact" analyses to an environmental impact study. This successful effort of the community planner to work with the planning board on the issue of the social impact of redevelopment involved the use of *negotiating* skills. The planner had to convince the planning board that the goals of physical and social planning were congruent, and that it was in the self-interest of the planning board to take into account both the social and the physical impact of housing redevelopment.

Facilitating Supportive Agency Environments

Community planners can facilitate supportive agency environments by providing technical consultation to human service organizations to assess the structures, functions and dynamics of these agencies. Through the use of such tools as the WES, planners provide organizational development consultation, assessing dysfunctional agency climates and recommending changes to administrators and staff. A measurement-feedback-planning process enables the consultant to highlight resistance to change, and purpose means for introducing innovations in light of the values and priorities of staff (Moos and Lemke 1983:159).

Societal Arena: Policy Analyst

The function of the social policy analyst is to formulate policies that lead to social support programming. These policies ensue from legislation on the local, state, and federal levels, as well as study commissions and executive-level planning departments on the state and federal levels. For example, the President's Commission on Mental Health (1978) recognized the importance of community support systems and social networks for service for the mentally ill. A federal initiative for funding community support systems has come from the National Institute of Mental Health (1977).

The discussion of the role of the policy analyst in the area of social support draws upon the framework presented in Chapter 1, which indicated that policy formulation is concerned with two major kinds of system change: changes in substantive goals and changes in strategies for achieving these goals.

Change in Substantive Goals

We have previously indicated that social support as a major intervention strategy can be directed at two different types of goals: prevention of social problems and service to persons who suffer from them. Changes in substantive goals occurs in four ways: (1) goal clarification; (2) shift in goal priorities; (3) addition of new goals; and (4) shift in mission.

Goal clarification, the process of assessing the relationship between goals and the means to achieve the goals, helps to avoid displacement of focus from ends to means. In formulating social support policies, the policy analyst reviews existing policies to evaluate (1) the extent to which the goals of social support are being achieved, and (2) the degree to which ends are being displaced by means to the detriment of the service user's benefit. For example, in the goal of balancing formal and informal care systems, the policy analyst will evaluate the extent to which formal service programs complement, supplement, or supplant natural helping networks (Warren 1981:210). This is accomplished by environmental impact analyses of efforts to integrate formal and informal care programs. If it is found that formal care systems are supplanting informal care, with negative consequences for the service user, then policies should be formulated to rectify this problem of goal displacement.

In the case situation, the policy analyst discovered that the goal of interweaving formal and informal care systems was not being accomplished, and that informal care was used as an excuse to withdraw formal care. The policy analyst recommended that the revised law specify that social support should be the preferred intervention to prevent institutional placement of the handicapped.

Shift in goal priorities involves changing the emphasis given to different goals. For example, if existing policy gives a higher priority to service than to prevention, and it is believed that preventive programs will result in greater benefits, then a new policy shifting the priority to prevention is indicated.

A third type of goal change is the *addition of new goals*. If evidence indicates that preventive interventions achieve positive results and these are not included in existing policy, then the addition of this new goal is indicated. In the case example, the new goal of prevention was recommended for inclusion in the revised statute.

Shift in mission means a major change in the direction of a program. An example of this is the change from traditional people-changing treatment services to environmentally oriented services related to social support. In the case, the recommendation was made to revise the law to include social support as the principle intervention in service to the handicapped.

As indicated in Chapter 1, the above types of goal changes vary in their feasibility. This has implications for the tasks required of the policy analyst. Since shifting of the mission from providing traditional treatment services to giving social support will require considerable pressure and power, the policy analyst will have to plan for the mobilization of this kind of support.

Change in Strategies for Achieving Goals

There are three types of change related to strategies for achieving goals: (1) internal structural change; (2) change in external relations; and (3) change in assessment of the results of program intervention.

Internal structural change refers to modifications in the kinds of organizational arrangements that agencies use to achieve their goals. Since there is some evidence that a participatory program structure facilitates community-oriented programs (Prager and Shnit 1985), policy formulation to achieve decentralization is indicated. Changes in staffing arrangements with emphasis on different professional roles and skills that are relevant for social support interventions is another area of internal structural change.

If current policies do not include a system of *objective assessment* as a strategy for monitoring program results, then the policy analyst formulate a new policy that provides for systematic procedures to evaluate program outcomes in terms of benefits to service users. In the case, it was evident that programming for the handicapped was evaluated in terms of effort rather than results. The policy analyst recommended a modification in the statute to include community maintenance as the basis for program evaluation.

Change in external relations refers to modifications in the open vs. closed nature of programs. As previously indicated, since social support goals require extensive interorganizational collaboration, among formal organizations as well as between formal and informal care systems, an open systems strategy is indicated. Therefore, a policy analyst will formulate policies that emphasize procedures for interorganizational cooperation, such as requiring affiliation agreements between institutions and aftercare programs stipulating community support services for persons discharged from residential care. In the case, lack of interagency coordination led to the recommendation to include a provision in the revised statute for a mechanism to facilitate interorganizational collaboration.

In the case, the tasks of the policy analyst cited above required that he have skill in *decision making.* Thus, in the goal clarification process, he had to first formulate the *problem* as to why the state statute was not accomplishing its goal of interweaving formal and informal care systems. He *searched for alternative solutions* to this problem and then made a decision as to what solution would solve this problem after evaluating the *cost* vs. *benefits* of the different alternatives. A similar decision-making procedure applies to the other goal-changing strategies, i.e., addition of goals and changing the mission. Decision-making skills were also needed in the decision to change the strategies for achieving social support goals.

INTEGRATION OF MICRO AND MACRO SOCIAL SUPPORT

As indicated in previous chapters on community resource coordination, micro and macro social support practice are interdependent. Practitioners on both levels should be aware of each other's practice roles and responsibilities. Micro practitioners should appreciate the need for administrative, planning, and policy support for their efforts. Likewise, macro practitioners depend on feedback from micro level line staff about the problems in implementing social support programs in order to make policies more functional.

SUMMARY

This chapter presented the macro aspects of social support interventions, examining the roles of administrator, planner, and policy analyst. Several issues related to the implementation of social support policy were discussed. The intervention roles of administrators of direct-service agencies were linked to three stages of organizational innovation. The community planner role was concerned with influencing the climate of community life through intervention in informal caring networks. The potential for community planners to enhance community life was also related to opportunities for integrating social and physical planning. A policy analysis model was then presented and applied to the social support area. Material from a case presented at the beginning of the chapter was used to illustrate the various macro intervention roles. Case material was also used to illustrate how practice skills are related to macro level social support interventions.

STUDY QUESTIONS

1. You have been hired as a management consultant by the Central County Association of Aging (CCAA) to help them redesign their organizational structure to better achieve social support goals. Which aspects of structure would you recommend changing first and why?

2. The administrator of CCAA asks your advice on whether the agency should give priority to preventive programs or use its resources for service users who have existing problems. Show how you would use the decision-making procedure to develop recommendations for this administrator.

3. You are a supervisor at the CCAA and are having difficulty persuading a subordinate that he needs to learn social support intervention skills. He was educated to do counseling and does not think social support is appropriate or effective for the disabled elderly. How would you influence this staff member to change his behavior? What skills would you use?

4. You are the person in charge of the newly created resource development unit in CCAA. With which agencies would you develop affiliation agreements to enhance the achievement of social support goals?

5. You are the community planner trying to develop an agreement with the planning board to integrate physical and social planning. How would you approach this task? What kind of skills would you need to use?

6. You are a legislative aide to a U.S. senator. He asks you to draft a bill on social support for the severely mentally ill. Using the policy framework included in Chapter 1, indicate what the basic elements of this plan would be?

Chapter 8

ORGANIZATIONAL ENVIRONMENTS

Organizational Environments

B. Behavior Settings
  1. Organizational Level Interventions
    a. Direct Service
    b. Administration
  2. Community Level Interventions
    a. Social Advocacy
    b. Community Planning
  3. Societal Level Interventions
    a. Social Policy Analysis
C. Organizational Structures
  1. Organizational Level Interventions
    a. Direct Service
    b. Administration
  2. Community Level Interventions
    a. Social Advocacy
    b. Community Planning
  3. Societal Level Interventions
    a. Policy Analyst
D. Staff and Service Consumer Culture
  1. Organizational Level Interventions
    a. Direct Service
    b. Administration
  2. Community Level Interventions
    a. Social Advocacy
    b. Community Planning
  3. Societal Level Interventions
    a. Social Policy Analysis
E. Organizational Climates
  1. Organizational Level Interventions
    a. Direct Service
    b. Administration
  2. Community Level Interventions
    a. Social Advocacy
    b. Community Planning
  3. Societal Level Interventions
    a. Social Policy Analysis

INTRODUCTION

Organizational environments have significant impact on professional practice. The physical and social characteristics of organizations, reflected in their structures, cultures, climates, and behavior settings, have been found to influence the functioning of service users and staff (Moos 1974a). For example, in hospital discharge planning, organizational factors overide professional characteristics (nurses vs. social workers) in determining staff activity (Iglehart 1990). Optimal functioning of professional staff requires an understanding of the opportunities and constraints that this agency environment has on their practice (Neugeboren 1991).

Micro and macro practitioners use knowledge of organizational environments to facilitate their practice. Direct-service staff employ this knowledge in making decisions on service consumer referrals to insure that the target agency's environment can meet individual service user's needs. Assessment of organizational environments is also important for administrators, planners, social advocates, and policymakers. Direct-service agency administrators must evaluate their agency's environments to determine whether they enhance or detract from service consumers' benefit. Organizational barriers to service effectiveness compel the administrator to take action to remedy these defects. Community planners also determine whether organizational environmental factors are facilitating or hindering effective service to service users. In their role of allocating funds to direct-service agencies, they can be instrumental in influencing organizational arrangements to enhance program outcomes. Community organizers who engage in user advocacy work with service consumer groups to remedy dysfunctional agency environments. Those formulating policies on the legislative level also must take into account how organizational environmental factors hinder or enhance the achievement of policy goals.

This chapter begins with a case situation of a handicapped individual receiving care in a nursing home. This case is used as a vehicle for illustrating how the organization's environment affects practice and service user benefit. Next, several issues will be discussed to highlight how the organization impacts on service-delivery practice. Five aspects of organizational environments will then be defined and discussed:

(1) physical environments; (2) behavior settings; (3) organizational climates; (4) structures; and (5) cultures. This knowledge will then be related to practice interventions in direct service, administration, planning and social advocacy, and policy formulation. The applicability of practice skills and the integration of micro and macro practice to organizational environmental situations follows. The chapter concludes with study questions to aid the reader in applying this knowledge of organizational environmental to practice situations.

CASE: COUNTY CONVALESCENT CENTER

Mrs. S

This situation is a continuation of the case of Mrs. S described in Chapter 6. After Mr. S' death, Mrs. S lived in her apartment for about five years, until she had a stroke and was placed at the county convalescent center (CCC). Prior to the stroke, she became increasingly depressed and stayed in bed, despite the efforts of a home health aide, her daughter and the social worker at the family agency to convince her that this was bad for her well-being. She also became socially isolated as she refused to leave her apartment.

Mrs. S was initially hospitalized in a general medical hospital after the stroke. Although the stroke was relatively minor, she did not respond to treatment and her condition deteriorated. She became quite depressed and said that she wanted to die. She received treatment from a variety of doctors, including an internist, neurologist, and psychiatrist. She complained that she was being used for experimentation (e.g., she was tested with brain scan). She refused to eat and had to be force-fed. At the end of the 30-days hospitalization that was covered by her insurance, she was discharged to the CCC.

County Convalescent Center

Physical Characteristics

The CCC is a recently built county-operated nursing home. The administrator of the facility was hired prior to its construction and was actively involved in the architectural planning for the building. The CCC is located about two miles from the area where Mrs. S had her apartment. It is accessible to the daughter by public transportation. It is in an urban area in proximity to other community programs such as religious services, and the nursing home provides transportation to these services.

The CCC is a 100-bed nursing facility. It is a four-story building with offices and a dining area and kitchen on the first floor. The remaining floors contain approximately 30 beds each. Since there are three patients in each room, each floor has approximately ten patient rooms. These rooms are located in proximity to the nursing station. In general, staff work well together and are attentive to the patients' needs. This physical layout of the home results in close proximity of the patients to each other and much social interaction.

The particular architectural design of the home caused much controversy. County officials waged a campaign to change the design to a more typical one, consisting of single-story building, which they thought would facilitate more-efficient management. Also, having three patients to a room was frowned on because of lack of patient privacy. The administrator hired to run this home was trained in social work administration and had many years experience as a nursing home administrator. She was convinced that the traditional architectural designs were dysfunctional because they isolated patients. The administrator overcame the opposition to this architectural plan by mobilizing support from the patient advocate in the County Office on Aging.

Integration vs. Segregation of Patients

The policy of the home is to integrate the senile with the mentally competent patients. Although Mrs. S' daughter found it upsetting to see her mother intermingled with the senile patients, Mrs. S did not seem to mind. The more-competent patients set high expectations for the senile ones and the latter responded positively to these demands. Also, the staff pressured the more competent patients to participate in their therapy by pointing to the more disabled patients as examples of what would happen if they did not cooperate.

The relatives of the nonsenile patients who opposed the policy of patient integration pressured the executive director to segregate these two groups of patients. They contacted their representatives on the county council urging them to exert influence to change the policy of integrating senile and nonsenile patients at the CCC.

The executive of the CCC waged a campaign to counteract the pressure of the relatives. She spoke with the community planner at the County Office on Aging and the policy analyst at the State Office of Medical Assistance, which funded nursing-home care. She stressed the positive value for service consumer benefit of the policy of integrating the more-competent and less-competent patients. She was also helped by support from a community organizer in the County Office on Aging who had received complaints from relatives of service users placed in segregated nursing homes. As a result, the integration policy was continued at the CCC. The publicity generated by this situation also induced the policy analyst in the State Office of Medical Assistance to pressure for a review of its regulations for nursing homes, resulting in changes supporting the integration of senile and nonsenile patients.

Patient and Staff Characteristics

At the time of the controversy, the staff of CCC consisted of administration, trained nurses, a social worker, the physical therapist, social activities person, nursing aides, and maintenance personnel. The center provided intensive nursing care for severely disabled persons. Since most of the staff were medically oriented, they did not appreciate the impact that the physical and social environment of the agency had on residents. To compensate for this deficiency, the administrator had the social worker conduct an in-service training program that focused on how environmental factors impinge on patient welfare. A staff performance evaluation system was also developed that took into account environmental practice accomplishment.

Although most of the patients in the CCC were severely disabled and required intensive care, there were some who were ambulatory and did not require this kind of service. They needed placement in a program that was appropriate for their higher level of functioning. The director did an annual assessment of the agency's environment, which revealed that these higher-level patients were inappropriately placed. Subsequently, she negotiated an agreement with a sheltered-care apartment complex in the area for referral of some of the higher-level ambulatory patients. The community planner from the County Office on Aging helped facilitate the promulgation of this affiliation agreement between the CCC and the sheltered-care apartment complex for referral of service consumers from CCC. The agreement required the CCC to reciprocate by accepting residents from the sheltered-housing complex who required nursing-home care.

Daily Routine

The daily routine was that *all* patients were required to spend their days out of bed participating in activities appropriate for their needs. Each floor had a room with a TV that many patients watched. The mentally competent patients congregated and socialized in the area near the front entrance of the building, where they also met with their visitors. Various recreational activities were planned, including arts and crafts, music, and special celebrations around holidays and birthdays.

Mrs. S' initial reaction to the routine was anger, particularly at her having to get out of bed every day. In general, Mrs. S resented the various rules and the firmness with which the head nurse enforced them. She expressed her resentment openly to the staff and referred to the head nurse as a "sergeant." After several weeks in the nursing home, Mrs. S' depression lifted, she regained her appetite, and she smiled for the first time in many months. She participated in social programs at the nursing home, particularly the socializing with other patients, as well as attending religious services in the community.

As Mrs. S' depression lifted, she expressed an interest in visiting with the people from the neighborhood where she previously lived. The head nurse (the sergeant!) refused to give permission. The nurses at the home discouraged residents from visiting in the community because they thought it would interfere with adjustment in the nursing home. Mrs. S. spoke with the social worker at the CCC, who was thoroughly familiar with the rules and regulations of the home, since she had worked there for many years. The social worker knew that the rules of the nursing home *did* allow for this kind of visiting; however, she had to be careful not to antagonize the head nurse, who had considerable power and influence. She spoke to the executive director and obtained permission for Mrs. S to visit her old neighborhood. She explained to the head nurse that Mrs. S was visiting with her son, which was true, since the son took her to visit her old neighborhood.

ISSUES

There are two issues related to the use of knowledge of organizational environments in practice. They are (1) can practitioners influence organizational environments? and (2) can environmental assessments be institutionalized?

Can Practitioners Influence Organizational Environments?

This chapter on organizational environments presupposes that practitioners can mediate the effects that an agency's environment has on their practice. The assumption is that by understanding the nature of this environment they can minimize the constraints and maximize the opportunities to enhance practice. Accomplishment of this goal requires having information on organizational environments. For example, a direct-service worker referring a service user needs information on the environments of target agencies in order to make a match with service consumer needs. Since this kind of data is not readily available, the worker should seek this out from those who have knowledge of these agencies. A resource coordination unit (see Chapter 4) can facilitate the collection of this kind of information.

Direct-service administrators, community planners, and policy analysts also need methods for obtaining information on organizational environments to determine if they need to be modified to achieve the goals of service user benefit. Macro practitioners have to master organizational innovation skills to change those agency environments that are dysfunctional for service consumers (Brager and Holloway 1978).

The availability of information on organizational environments is dependent on whether resources are allocated for the ongoing assessment of human-service agency environments. This will affect the feasibility of institutionalizing an agency environmental assessment, which is the next issue to be discussed.

Can Agency Environmental Assessments Be Institutionalized?

Given the proliferation of mandated external reviews in the human services, a way of institutionalizing environmental assessment would be to incorporate them as part of these reassessment procedures. The institutionalization of agency environmental assessments will require funding authorities to mandate them as a regular part of program evaluation and review. For example, many states require nursing homes to have periodic external reviews as part of the requirements for medicare and medicaid eligibility. The administration of an environmental assessment instrument such as the Multiphasic Environmental Procedure (MEAP) could be included as a routine part this external review. A similar requirement could be added for the accreditation of hospitals by the Joint Commission on Hospital Accreditation. State and local funding authorities could also mandate agency environmental assessments as a requirement in their requests for proposals.

The feasibility of including environmental assessments as part of external review procedures will in all likelihood be influenced by the extent to which they are perceived as relevant for service evaluation. The initiative for introducing this kind of assessment may be more feasible if done first on an individual agency basis. Thus, the leadership for this innovation may have to come from administrators of direct-service agencies. Support for the incorporation of environmental assessments as a regular part of external review requirements can also come from community organizers, planners, and policy analysts.

DEFINITIONS

The impact of organizational environments on service users has been systematically studied under the rubric of social ecology (Moos 1984). Scales have been developed to evaluate educational, treatment, family, and work environments (Moos 1974). This chapter's focus is on the impact that service agency environments have on service consumers. For some discussion of the effects of work and family environments on staff and family members see Chapter 6.

Five environmental areas that affect practice are: (1) physical environments; (2) behavior settings and expectations; (3) organizational structures; (4) staff and service user culture; and (5) organizational climates. These five areas of the physical and social environments will be applied to direct service, planning, community organization, and policy in the organizational, community, and societal arenas. The five areas are derived from the MEAP scale, which is an instrument that objectively measures these dimensions in institutional environments (Moos and Lemke 1984).

Physical Environments

The physical environment includes the architectural and geographical aspects of environmental intervention (Gutheil 1992). Among the relevant elements are community accessibility, physical features, physical aids, and space allowances. Accessibility relates to the proximity of the facility to resources in the surrounding community. Physical features include those that add convenience and comfort (physical amenities) or foster social interaction and recreational activities (e.g., social and recreational aids). Architectural features also can aid or hinder social interaction (e.g., long corridors foster service consumer isolation). Physical aids can enhance physical independence and mobility (prosthetic aids), visual cues to orient the resident (orientation aids), and such features as good lighting, nonskid surfaces on stairs and ramps, smoke detectors, and call buttons in bathrooms (safety features). Space allowances relate to the amount of space available for resident and staff functions.

In the case, the location of the nursing home on a public transportation route facilitated the access of Mrs. S' relatives. The multistory architecture of the nursing home allowed a small number of rooms on each floor (ten), resulting in short halls, close proximity of patients and staff and maximization of patient and staff, social interaction.

Behavior Settings and Expectations

Behavior settings are environmental factors that influence behavior expectations (Lamb and Goertzel 1972; Weinman and Kleiner

1978). Behavior settings fall into two categories. The first is the extent to which behavioral requirements are imposed on residents. This includes: (1) expectations for functioning–the minimum acceptable capacity to perform daily living tasks; and (2) tolerance for deviance–the extent to which uncooperative, aggressive, or eccentric behavior is tolerated.

The second category is the balance between individual freedom and institutional order and stability. Included here are such characteristics as the extent to which residents of an institution can select individual patterns of daily routine, and influence policy, the clarity with which that policies are communicated, and the amount of privacy available to residents.

Human service agencies have procedures for service users to participate in their governance. Mental hospitals have regular patient/staff meetings to discuss various problems arising in the operation of the agency. Nursing homes frequently arrange meetings with relatives of patients. These meetings provide feedback to administrators, resulting in changes in policies and procedures. Another strategy to achieve service consumer influence is the participation of service users on agency boards that make organizational policies.

In the case, it appears that the CCC stressed order, control, and stability, and provided a minimum of privacy (e.g., three patients to a room) and no formal structure for feedback from patients and relatives. With regard to Mrs. S, this controlled environment met her individual needs.

Organizational Structures

Organizational structures operate on both an official and an operative level. The *official* structure is the set of written rules and regulations. The operative structure is the behavior of staff in their daily activities. Both official and operative structures can affect practice. The effective micro and/or macro practitioner analyzes these structural influences in order to minimize their constraints and maximize the opportunities they present for practice to achieve service consumer benefit.

These patterns of staff behavior are guided by role, authority, communication, reward, and interorganizational structures. The role structure is the expected behavior of staff in the performance of particular organizational roles (e.g., direct-service worker, supervisor, administrator). The authority structure indicates who has the power to make decisions in the organization. The communication structure is the network for the dissemination of information in the agency. The reward structure is the system for allocating rewards and sanctions, such as promotions and dismissals. The interorganizational structure is the pattern of relations between the agency and other service organizations (Neugeboren 1991). (For additional discussion of organizational structure see Chapter 7.)

The absence of organizational structure can have negative effects on service users (Stanton and Schwartz 1954; York and Henley 1986:5). Small organizational size is associated with a greater service orientation of staff (Thomas 1959). The negative effects on service consumers who reside in "total institutions," which are very large, has been demonstrated (Goffman 1961). Decentralized structures are associated with better service user outcomes (Prager and Shnit 1985). In the case, the small size of the nursing home (100 patients) and the decentralization of the patients into three separate floors facilitated a service orientation. The centralized authority structure (e.g., head nurse) was functional for meeting Mrs. S' needs.

Culture of Staff and Service Consumers

The environment of any social unit is a function of its inhabitants, who bring to it values, norms and abilities. The attributes of the aggregate membership determine the subculture that develops, which in turn affects individual members. Several aspects of staff and service user characteristics have been identified: (1) staff characteristics; (2) characteristics of residents; and (3) resident functioning.

Staff characteristics reflect the resources available from staff in terms of experience and training. Resident characteristics relate to demographic variables that result in heterogeneity or homogeneity. Resident functioning refers to residents' independence in performing daily functions. The variation in functional ability of service consumers also determines service user diversity.

In the case, the nursing home was heterogeneous in terms of the level of functioning of the residents. The policy of intermingling of the patients had positive effects for both the lower and higher functioning patients.

Organizational Climates

Organizational climates are determined by the *perceptions* of staff and service consumers. The social climate framework consists of: (1) relationships—the extent of conflict or cohesion; (2) personal growth—the extent to which independence or dependence is encouraged; and (3) system flexibility—the extent to which stress is placed on order and control vs. service users feeling that they have the opportunity for participation and influence.

In the nursing home case, both staff and patients were cohesive in their relationships. Patient independence was encouraged in terms of the high expectations for their behavior. There was also stress on order and control, which as indicated previously, facilitated Mrs. S' progress.

INTERVENTIONS

The discussion of interventions in organizational environments examines micro and macro practice roles in the organizational, community, and societal arenas in the five organizational environmental areas just discussed. It will be followed by the presentation of a general intervention model, using a systematic approach to monitoring and feedback of the results of organizational assessments to improve agency functioning. The roles performed by micro and macro practitioners will then be highlighted to show the linkage with the conceptual framework presented in Chapter 1.

Physical Environments

The physical environment includes the geographical and architectural aspects of environmental practice. Practice that takes into account the physical environment is concerned with community accessibility and how physical features of the agency impinge on the needs of service users.

Organizational Level Interventions

Direct Service. Direct-service staff use information on functional and dysfunctional physical environments to make service consumer referral decisions. Case managers do assessments of individual physical environmental needs that result in referral to services that provide these particular environmental resources. For example, if a service consumer requires services from several community agencies, it is important that each facility to which the service user is being referred is physically accessible. In the case, the CCC was located in an area that was in close proximity to other community services.

Administration. Administrative responsibility for the design of organizational structures also applies to planning physical environments so as to enhance service consumer functioning. Administrators of direct-service agencies who are involved in the design of new facilities should influence architectural planning to enhance resident social interaction (e.g., minimizing long corridors). Similarly, should the geographic location of a new agency facilitate physical accessibility to relatives and to community services (e.g., location near public transportation).

In the case, the administrator of the nursing home successfully influenced the design of the structure of the agency to meet the needs of the service users being served. The multistory design of this nursing home facilitated social interaction of patients and staff by minimizing long corridors and maximizing close proximity of patient rooms.

Community Level Interventions

Social Advocacy. Community interventions on the micro level take into account how architectural factors affect service consumer benefit. Community organizers use information obtained from service users to mobilize support for more functional architectural design of agency physical structures. In the case, the opposition to the controversial architectural design used in planning the CCC was overcome with the help of the patient advocate in the County Office on Aging.

Community Planning. Community-planning intervention in relation to physical environments also involves influencing direct service agencies to develop benevolent physical environments for their programs. For example, a county human-service planner doing needs assessments and making decisions on the allocation of funds should include in the request for proposals that geographic and architectural factors be considered. Priority should be given to those programs that are physically accessible to those community agencies with which its service consumers are to be linked. Architectural features could also be included in the criteria for *monitoring* and allocation of capital funds.

Societal Level Interventions

Social Policy Analysis. Policy formulation involving physical environmental factors focuses on strategies for achievement of *system goals.* Specifically, attention is given to national and state policies that establish parameters for social programs, taking these factors into account. Here again, policies should be established to promote the construction of facilities that have more benevolent physical environments and are geographically located to facilitate accessibility. Social policy that encourages co-location of agency services would facilitate service user accessibility to these services.

Since housing is a critical need for many service consumer groups, such as the severely disabled being discharged from institutions, state and federal policies should take into account how architecture can influence service user well-being. Policy analysts need to be knowledgeable about the different types of housing required by the disabled (e.g., congregate housing for the elderly, transitional housing for those requiring a more supportive environment following discharge from an institution, small group homes for the developmentally disabled, and different types of sheltered-care facilities for the severely disabled).

The case illustrates the need to examine federal and state policies for the care of the elderly in the community and in institutions. The biases of funding programs such as medicare for institutional-based programs probably resulted in Mrs. S being kept in the hospital longer than necessary. To rectify this problem, policy analysts on the national level need to develop proposals for changing the regulations governing medicare.

Legislation that funds construction of health facilities such as nursing homes should be influenced by social policy analysts to use an architectural design similar to that of the nursing home in the case. One-story buildings that require long corridors, resulting in social isolation of patients. These should be discouraged in favor of taller buildings, which have fewer rooms on each floor and more opportunity for patient social interaction.

Behavior Settings

Behavior settings reflect the behavior expectations and behavior limits of service consumers, including expectation for functioning, levels of deviance tolerated, the balance between service user freedom and the organization's need for order and stability, and the extent to which service consumers can influence agency policy.

Organizational Level Interventions

Direct Service. Direct-service practitioners on the organizational level takes into account different behavior settings in referral of service users. Case managers need to plan for the progressive movement of service consumers from settings with different expectation levels. Ideally, one would expect that service users would move progressively to less-controlled settings. This occurs for service consumers discharged from institutions to transitional residences to prepare them for more autonomous functioning in the community (*normalized environments*). The reverse would occur for service users who are expected to diminish in social functioning over time (e.g., the elderly).

A worker assessment of Mrs. S' situation in her apartment (see case in Chapter 6) would have indicated that it was a low-expectation environment that was not suited for her needs. The daughter and case aide could not create the structure needed by Mrs. S. Her social isolation associated with living alone in an apartment was another problem. The family service worker might have considered a referral to a supervised congregate-living situation that would have alleviated this isolation and perhaps prevented Mrs. S' depression and subsequent stroke. With this type of service consumer, whose condition might deteriorate over time behavioral settings with increasing structure will be needed as the ability to function autonomously decreases. "Continuous care retirement communities" (Weeden 1986) are agencies that provide for this kind of continuum of care.

Administration. Macro interventions in behavior settings involve administrative formulations of policies that prescribe what is expected from service users. These policies should be consistent with the needs of those served. Policy decisions concerning the extent to which service consumers have freedom, choice, and control as members of the organization vs. the needs of the agency for stability and order are critical ones. Intrinsic to the establishment of these policies are *organizational-design* decisions, involving the creation of structures that will insure that staff will be able to function to meet the needs of service consumers. These decisions would range from establishing procedures for responding to service user deviancy to setting the boundaries of service consumers' power to collectively influence agency policies (Hasenfeld 1983). Service user influence of agency policies can be accomplished by the establishment of service consumer/staff meetings to obtain feedback from service users on procedures and policies that are not meeting their needs and therefore have to be changed. Another approach administrators can use enhance service consumer influence is to have them participate as agency board members.

The case illustrates how the policy of this agency provided the high behavior expectations required by Mrs. S. It should be noted that Mrs. S' anger at the firm application of rules helped to lift her depression.

Community Level Interventions

Social Advocacy. Social advocacy for groups of service users to promote functional behavior settings falls within the province of community organizers and public advocates for the disabled. Community organizers who work with service consumers are in a position to appreciate their potential for a higher level of functioning than is assumed by many human service professionals. This includes their potential for assuming the role of agency board members. These social advocates can enhance service user influence by making this information available to community planners, administrators, and policymakers in order to correct errors of underestimating service consumers abilities and capacities.

In the case, the collective need of the nursing home residents for a behavior setting that allowed social integration of patients with different levels of functioning was evident to the community organizer at the County Office on Aging, who successfully represented this to the authorities. This illustrates a policy that supports a toleration of deviance over the organizations need for control.

The lack of opportunity for patient and/or relative participation in the governance of this agency provides the opening for a community organizer to exert pressure to induce the administration to develop such a program.

Community Planning. Community planners also influence the behavior expectations of human service programs. They plan programs with varying behavioral expectations to meet the needs of different service user groups. For example, service consumers that are capable of semiautonomous functioning require settings that facilitate their independence (e.g., halfway houses). Different expectation settings are required to meet the changing needs of service users. Evidence suggests that human service programs tend to underestimate the ability of service consumers to assume control of their lives and to make decisions (Fairweather 1969).

Planners should include this variable of differential behavior settings in accordance with varying service users wants in their *needs assessment* studies. An example might be the assessment of the relationship between acute-care general hospital services and nursing-home programs for the severely disabled. Acute services, which provide emergency treatment, will have low behavior expectations of patients, who are passive recipients of service. In contrast, behavior expectations in long-term care agencies should strive for maximization of resident functioning. In this arena of medical care, planners should facilitate affiliation agreements between general hospitals and nursing homes that take into account these differences in behavior expectation environments associated with service consumers' needs. The promotion of high-expectation environments can be a force that influences severely disabled service users to function at maximum levels.

Community health planners could learn from the above case of the inappropriateness of the services of the acute-care general hospital in meeting the needs of this frail elderly individual. Equipped to treat acute illness with the intensive use of lifesaving medical technologies, general hospitals are not able to provide the supportive environment needed by the frail elderly as well as a facility designed for long-term care. Health planners need to take into account these factors in the criteria used for issuing certificates of need required for hospital construction. In the case situation, it probably was unnecessary for Mrs. S to remain in the hospital for the one-month period covered by her insurance.

The case also illustrated the role that can be assumed by the community planner in *facilitating coordination between agencies* with different behavior expectations. The planner facilitated an affiliation agreement between the nursing home and sheltered-care apartments.

Community planners can increase service consumer participation in agency governance by including this expectation in requests for proposals for program funding.

Societal Level Interventions

Social Policy Analysis. Social policy analysts formulate state and national policies that provide for different types of behavior expectation settings. This relates to changes in *internal strategies for achievement of substantive* goals. Specifically, change in behavior settings is associated with modification of internal structures. A case in point is the policy of medicare funding, which emphasizes treatment in acute-service general hospitals. As indicated, acute-treatment facilities have low behavior-expectation environments, with the consequence that patients with chronic conditions are unable to receive the social care appropriate for their needs.

In the case situation, Mrs. S' insurance coverage for hospitalization was used before she was referred to a nursing home. Her physical and mental deterioration in the low behavior-expectation environment of the hospital was reversed after she was placed in the high-expectation milieu of the nursing home. The policy analyst in the State Office of Medical Assistance utilized this knowledge in supporting a change in state policy of integration of senile and nonsenile patients, illustrating how this type of professional can help promote behavior settings that are relevant for service user needs.

Policy analysts, influence service user authority through legislation and regulations requiring client participation on agency boards.

Organizational Structures

Organizational structures are the relatively stable patterns of staff activities that reflect role expectations, the distribution of power, communication networks, reward systems, and the relations with other agencies.

Organizational Level Interventions

Direct Service. Direct-service practitioners within organizations must know how structure can constrain or facilitate their work with service consumers. Although rules are intrinsic to practice in formal organizations, staff have the discretion to interpret these rules for the benefit of service users. Given the problems endemic to providing individualized services in large bureaucratic systems, the direct-service worker needs to analyze the opportunities for using the structure to achieve service consumer benefit. Detailed knowledge of the rules (e.g., service manual) can provide the experienced worker with options for obtaining service which may not be readily apparent to the novice.

Case managers coordinating services for users between different agencies need to be sensitive to how boundary (turf) differences can constrain their efforts. This comes from the understanding of *inter-organizational structure.* Direct-service staff doing case coordination should understand how cooperation and conflict between agencies influence their practice. Their day-to-day problems in doing case coordination can be a useful source of information to community planners and administrators, alerting them to the need for systematic case and program coordination (see chapters 4 and 5 on community resource coordination). In the case, the affiliation agreement between the CCC and the sheltered-care apartment complex facilitated coordination between these two agencies.

The way in which knowledge of rules enables her to use the structure is illustrated in the case. The social worker, knowing the rules and regulations of the nursing home and aware of the power of the head nurse (operative power structure), was able to obtain official approval for Mrs S to visit her old neighbor without antagonizing the "sergeant."

Administration. Macro organizational interventions to influence structure require administrators of direct-service agencies to formulate policies that create role, authority, communication, reward, and interorganizational structures that enhance service consumer benefit. The *design of organizational structures* by administrators will be influenced by the knowledge that nonhierarchical participatory structures and small organizational size facilitate positive service user outcomes. Administrators need to weigh the balance between the value of decentralization of authority and the need for centralized controls to achieve service consumer benefit.

Administrators, who are required to create organizational structures in human service organizations, have to deal with professional resistance to formalized rules and procedures. Professionals often assume that structure will limit their freedom and autonomy (Neugeboren 1991). Administrators need to educate staff to recognize that structure provides boundaries for behavior, which facilitates professional autonomy. More important, the lack of structure can lead to such problems as role conflict and increased personal control by superiors (Rosengren 1967).

In the case, the director appreciated the need to use the *role structure* to support the social worker's efforts to facilitate Mrs. S' visit to her old neighborhood. However, the director also was aware of the *authority structure* (i.e., the power of the head nurse) and the importance of not challenging her. The development of a staff performance evaluation system is an example of the creation of a *reward structure.*

The administrator also was responsible for the agency's policy of integrating the senile and nonsenile service users. This facilitated staff and patient interactions. This is an illustration of the creation of a *communication structure.* When this policy was challenged by the relatives, the director mobilized support from the county and state, which relates to use of an *interorganizational structure.*

Community Level Interventions

Social Advocacy. Community organizers should know how *interorganizational structure* influences their practice. In their representation of service consumer needs to community agencies, they have to be cognizant of the official and unofficial linkages between organizations. They also should be aware of community power structures in order to utilize their influence.

Community Planning. Community planners, in doing *needs assessments, interorganizational coordination, and monitoring and feedback,* should take into account such structural factors as organizational size of allocating funds. The current trend of organizational mergers to achieve more efficiency should be examined in terms of the consequences to service users, who are not necessarily better served by larger and more complex systems. Also, the absence of structure in professionalized agencies might be examined to determine if there are negative effects on service consumers. If this lack is detrimental to service user benefit, then allocating agencies may need to establish more specific criteria for decisions for granting funds based on structural standards.

Planners operating on the community level are directly involved in the *interorganizational structure* area. As human service agencies become increasingly dependent on each others services, such interorganizational arrangements as affiliation agreements are developed to formalize the exchange of needed resources. Community planners can promote *interagency coordination* by influencing the *communication structure* (e.g., by facilitating discussion between agencies to increase their awareness of their interdependencies). Planners can promote interorganizational cooperation by helping human service agencies to become aware of the commonality of goals and opportunities for resource exchange (Reid 1965). This function for community planners, which involves the *role structure* of planning organizations, can help alleviate "turf" conflicts that are endemic between agencies. In the case, the community planner facilitated the development of an affiliation agreement between the CCC and the sheltered-care apartment complex.

Societal Level Interventions

Policy Analyst. Policy analysts on the state and federal levels should appreciate the effect that structure has on *strategies for achievement of program goals.* Although details of program implementation are usually not prescribed in legislation, consideration should be given to whether such conditions as interorganizational agreements and decentralized structures should be included. Given the complexity of social problems, requiring multiagency collaboration would seem to be justified.

Success in enacting legislation which requires collaboration between different constituent groups is also dependent on an understanding of *interorganizational structure.* In order to be successful in mobilizing support for legislation, policy analysts should know which agency interdependencies could be used to gain constituency support.

The size of the nursing home in the case (100 beds) facilitated effective service delivery. A policy analyst advising on criteria for funding nursing-home construction should take into account the structural factor of organizational size.

Policy analysts working for central offices of human service agencies use the understanding of interorganizational structure to institutionalize affiliation agreements between agencies serving the same service consumers by mandating this in state regulations. This would apply to such interdependent organizations as mental hospitals and community mental health centers; public assistance and child protection organizations; correctional institutions and probation and parole agencies and health and welfare organizations. This policy intervention recognizes that the need for greater cooperation between human service agencies is based on *open systems strategy* in policy formulation. In the case, this would have mandated the affiliation agreement between the CCC and the sheltered-care apartment complex.

Staff and Service Consumer Culture

As indicated previously, staff and service consumer culture reflects the values, norms, and abilities of the staff and service users.

Organizational Level Interventions

Direct Service. The direct-service worker within an agency needs to be aware of the impact that staff and resident characteristics have on their practice. If a characteristic of staff is to downplay professionalism because they are made up mostly of nonprofessionals (e.g., hospital aides, prison guards), then the professionally educated direct-service worker will have to take this into account in setting service goals.

Nursing homes and hospitals have a culture dominated by the medical and nursing professions. These professions may stress the value of in-patient service and minimize links with the community. The social worker in the case situation took this into account in developing strategies to deal with the head nurse in order to help Mrs. S maintain contacts with her old neighbors.

In the case, the culture of service users in the nursing home was a function of the characteristics of the patients in the CCC, which consisted of a mixture of high and low functioning patients. This culture was linked to the practice of integrating senile and nonsenile patients, which created a high-expectation environment. A direct-service worker would use such information in helping service consumers to maximize their functioning.

Case managers and discharge planners also need to know about the different cultural milieus of other agencies with which they are working. Their individual case planning takes into account the needs of the service user and how the organizational cultures of different agencies match these needs. For example, if they are working with a low-functioning severely mentally ill service user who they think would benefit from a high-expectation milieu, they should refer the user to an agency that integrates service consumers without reard to level of functioning. In the case, higher-functioning patients were referred to an agency (sheltered-care apartments) that had an environment requiring more-independent behavior.

Administration. Administrators of direct-service agencies should understand the impact that the characteristics of staff and residents have on the creation of the culture and milieu of their agencies, and how this particular environment impacts *goal formulation, design of organizational structures, and program implementation.* For example, if staff are professionals whose training stressed service to acutely disturbed patients (e.g., physicians, nurses, psychologists, etc.), then the official goals of programs for the severely disabled may not be congruent with their professional training. *Goal formulation* enables the administrator to be cognizant of how the particular resident culture fits the staff culture in the establishment of agency goals. Goal formulation will then influence the *design of organizational structures* in influencing the staff *roles*. This will affect the planning for the recruitment, selection, and in-service training of staff.

Admission policies, which relate to the *program implementation*, will be influenced by whether service consumer heterogeneity or homogeneity is more desirable in terms of the goals of the program. Should admission policy select primarily acutely disturbed service users or a mixture of both acute and severely disabled service consumers? How will a mix of acute and severely disabled patients affect the staff recruitment policies and the cohesiveness of staff? Will the selection of staff to work with these two different groups result in there being two distinct staff groups with different ideological orientations geared to two different organizational goals (e.g., social care for theseverely disabled vs. rehabilitation for the acutely disabled), with the consequence of ideological wars?

In a nursing home, should the lower-functioning patients be segregated or mainstreamed (Aviram and Segal 1973) with higher-functioning service users? What will be the effect of integration on these two kinds of patients? What will the consequence be for efficient allocation of staff manpower if patients are integrated or segregated? In the case, the CCC provided an organizational culture that was congruent with Mrs. S' needs. The patient culture consisted of a mix of senile and nonsenile patients. This was used by staff to support a high-expectation environment that met the needs of both the high and low functioning patients.

Community Level Interventions

Social Advocacy. Service user advocates representing different groups of service consumers need to appreciate the diverse values, norms, and functioning of these groups. Values and norms will differ among various ethnic groups and social classes (Devore and Schlesinger 1981).

Community organizers working with self-help groups for the severely disabled are in a good position to represent their potentials for higher-level functioning than is often assumed possible by the public in general and by professionals in particular. In their advocacy role, community organizers can influence direct-service agency administrators, community planners, and policy analysts to have higher expectations of service consumers in the assessment or agency cultures.

Community Planning. Community planners concerned with service integration should collect information on the cultures of the different agencies they are coordinating. Since agency cultures correspond to agency goals, the lack of goal congruence between agencies can be a barrier to their working cooperatively together.

Decisions to allocate funds should also be influenced by an understanding of the milieus present in the organizations being funded. If assessment of community needs indicates that certain kinds of agency environmental milieus are lacking, then funding allocations should be directed so as to fill these needs. For example, there are a significant number of high-functioning patients in nursing homes who would be better served by more independent living arrangements, such as sheltered-care apartments. Community planners could address this need by allocating funds to shelterd-care institutions.

Societal Level Interventions

Social Policy Analysis. Goal clarification also requires an understanding of agency culture. Legislation directed at the establishment of comprehensive systems of services should take into account the diversity of agency cultures in relation to service user needs. If heterogeneity is desirable, then statutes establishing programs should emphasize general rather than specialized programs. For example, addiction programs should include services for alcoholics and drug addicts.

Organizational Climates

Social climates of organizations are associated with the extent of conflict or cohesion between service users, the impact the agency has on service consumer freedom and autonomy, and service users' opportunity to influence agency policies. Organizational climates are a product of the *perceptions* of service users and staff.

Organizational Level Interventions

Direct Service. Direct-service workers who match service consumer individual needs with environmental resources should determine if the social climate of an agency is or is not functional for their service users. The direct-service worker could feed this information back to administration in order to help shape policy to meet the needs of service consumers. Intake workers would need to determine if different programs in an agency have different social climates that may be appropriate for different types of service users. For example, it might be expected that an inpatient service would stress control more an outpatient program. This variation in climates between programs would provide the worker with the opportunity to utilize these services in a differential manner in accordance with the needs of service consumers.

In the case, the degree of control exerted by the head nurse might be seen by the direct-service worker as dysfunctional for the service users' need for freedom and autonomy. This was evident in the worker's action to circumvent the head nurse in facilitating Mrs. S' visit to her old neighborhood.

Case managers coordinating services for individual service consumers have to be aware of the variation in social climates among agencies. This information can be used to achieve a continuum of care for service users (e.g., making a plan for movement of a service consumer from a more to a less controlled environment such as from an institution to care in the community). This is illustrated in the case where ambulatory patients were transferred to sheltered-care apartments.

Administration. Administrators of direct-service agencies should know the extent to which their service users and staff perceive that the agency social climate is free vs. controlling; encourages dependence vs. independence; and is cohesive vs. conflict ridden. These perceptions are evaluated in terms of their congruence with the official goals of the agency. For example, if the agency serves adolescents who act out, then a certain amount of order and control may be functional. On the other hand, if the service consumers have been discharged from a custodial agency that has a low-expectation environment, a freer social climate may be indicated. In general, information on these social climate dimensions could be used as a guide by administrators to introduce organizational change through *goal clarification* that would modify social climates to make them congruent with the goals of the agency. In the case, the social climate of the CCC was a mixture of control and participation, which seemed appropriate for the goals of the agency.

Community Level Interventions

Social Advocacy. The fact that organizational climates are determined by the *perceptions* of service users places responsibility on community organizers, through their work with service consumer groups, to access this information and make it available to service users and professionals. Community organizers can systematically survey the perceptions of both current and past service consumers as to their experiences in the agencies where they received service. For example, service users involved with self-help groups for the mentally ill can be interviewed about their perceptions of their experience in mental institutions, specifically regarding the opportunity they had for participation and influence in the agency or the extent of conflict or cohesion in the agency. This data on organizational climates will need to be made available to community planners, who would be responsible for communicating it to administrators of direct service agencies.

Community Planning. Community planners could use these social climate dimensions as criteria for *needs assessment* studies. For example, a survey of key informants may determine that there is need for programs that foster service consumer independence, and this information could then be used to influence the allocation of funds. The MEAP scale could be used to evaluate the social climate of an agency that is being funded for a particular program, to determine if there is consistency between the purposes of the grant and the climate of the organization. As indicated above, community planners would also obtain information on agency climates from community organizers who work with service user groups.

Societal Level Interventions

Social Policy Analysis. Since organizational climates are a function of staff and service consumer perception, it would be difficult to affect climates through legislative mandate. If these climates were found to correlate with such factors as staff characteristics, then policies could be formulated establishing criteria for staff selection, which falls into the policy formulation area of *internal strategies for goal achievement.*

MODEL FOR SYSTEMATIC ASSESSMENT TO IMPROVE ORGANIZATIONAL ENVIRONMENTS

The use of environmental interventions in different areas of practice has been discussed above. Here we outline a more general approach to monitoring and improving agency environments. Using the MEAP Scale, administrators and staff can better understand their organizational ecology for purposes of clarifying goals and introducing facility modifications to better meet the needs of service users. Moos and Lemke (1984) suggest the following four steps for environmental change: (1) environmental assessment, (2) feedback of the results of assessment, (3) planning and instituting change, and (4) reassessment.

The MEAP profiles on several dimensions can point to where change could be most readily and effectively initiated (Moos, Lemke, and Clayton 1983). Feedback of environmental assessments to staff can help motivate them to cooperate in organizational change efforts. Data from the assessment process can be used in staff training and development by defining administrator and staff roles and identifying organizational sanction and sources of resistance to change. Moos and Lemke (1984:75) note that

> The assessment-feedback process may prepare a facility for later modifications by clarifying the conceptual framework of administrators and staff, giving staff members a common language for discussing their setting, and encouraging staff to adopt the role of program designer and planner.

In the case, feedback of the organizational assessment led to an in-service training program for staff.

Practice Skills Applied to Organizational Environments

Decision Making

As indicated previously, micro and macro practitioners use knowledge of organizational environments to make case and policy decisions. In case practice, the decision-making process, which includes the *formulation of a service consumer's problem* and the determination of appropriate alternative solutions, should evaluate the fit between individual need and the available environmental resources. For example, in deciding where to refer Mrs. S, the hospital social worker used information on the service user's behavior in the hospital setting to arrive at a plan for referral to a setting that had the structure and behavior expectations appropriate for her needs. The worker, in seeking an appropriate setting for Mrs. S, may have compared several nursing homes in terms of their physical and social environments. The *evaluation of these alternatives* led her to the decision that the *cost/benefit* ratio of these alternative nursing homes in terms of meeting Mrs. S' need justified the decision to place her at the CCC.

The *nonrational factors* in the decision-making process also needed to be considered in the referral decision. Pressure was exerted by the hospital to have Mrs. S discharged by the end of her 30-day insurance coverage. This pressure from the hospital administration probably precluded a complete search for a nursing home that could provide her with the "best" environment to meet her needs.

Monitoring

In addition to the practice skill in decision making, micro and macro professionals also need to use monitoring skills to determine if organizational environments are functional for service consumer needs. For example, in the case the administrator evaluated the physical and social environment of the CCC to determine if it was congruent with the resident's needs. This evaluation determined that there were service users who required a more independent living arrangement. This led to the formulation of an agreement to have them transferred to a sheltered-care apartment complex.

Community organizers working with service consumer groups also use monitoring skills in assembling information from service users on their perception of organizational climates.

The monitoring skill is used by community planners to determine if the agencies they are funding are providing the kind of environments required by service consumerss. In the case, the expectation setting of the general hospital should have been monitored to determine if it was appropriate for the kinds of patients being served. If this hospital serves many elderly and other severely disabled, as is often the case, then the planning agency should take steps to influence the hospital to do more expeditious discharge planning to settings that have behavior expectations that are appropriate for this type of patient.

Negotiating

Negotiating skills are used to achieve coordination between and within organizations. As indicated previously, collaboration between agencies that have different physical and social environments will be affected by the interdependency between these organizations in terms of these social-ecological environmental factors. For example, an interdependency exists between low behavior expectation/high-structure institutional settings and high expectation/low-structure community settings in the achievement of a continuum of care. Goal interdependence is used by practitioners as the basis for negotiating agreements between different agencies. This is illustrated in the case in the relationship between the CCC and the sheltered-care apartment complex.

Representing

Representing skills are used by practitioners to market their programs in terms of their unique environmental characteristics. Such characteristics as physical environments that facilitate service user interaction, high behavior expectation settings, heterogeneous service user mix, etc., should be used in public relations programs to market agency services to consumers and referral organizations. This kind of marketing took place in the case, where the administrator of CCC represented her agency in the negotiations with the sheltered-care apartment complex.

Staffing

Staffing skills, which include personnel recruitment, selection, training, evaluation, and establishment of reward systems, are also necessary for effective work in organizational environments. Staff who are skilled in assessing the impact of organizational environments on service consumers need to be selected and trained. Those professionals who lack these skills should receive training to make up for this deficit. In the case, it was evident that the medically oriented nursing staff was not sympathetic to the value of having Mrs. S maintain her contacts with neighbors from the community in which she had previously lived. An in-service training program was instituted to remedy this skill deficiency.

INTEGRATION OF MICRO AND MACRO PRACTICE

The integration of micro and macro practice in this area of organizational environments is based on the need for communication between these level of practice. Communication is required in both directions: from direct service practitioners, community organizers to administrators, planners and policy analysts as well as from macro to micro practitioners.

Communication from Micro to Macro Practitioners

Direct-service practitioners, through their involvement with service users, are in a position to obtain information on organizational environments. They can communicate service consumers perceptions of whether particular agency environments are functional or dysfunctional for their needs. This information can help administrators of direct-service agencies to assess the environments of their particular organizations and determine any changes that are needed. This information can also be useful for community planners in their task of doing needs assessments, facilitating interagency coordination, and monitoring. Policy analysts will also be able to use this information in formulating social policies.

Communication from Macro to Micro Practitioners

Administrators and planners who assess organizational environments in the performance of their responsibilities can be a useful source of information to direct-service practitioners. Direct-service agencies can include information on organizational environments in their centralized community-resource data banks for use by direct practitioners employed in these organizations. Community-planning agencies that collect information on community resources can also include information on organizational environments to be made available to direct-service practitioners through resource directories.

SUMMARY

The following list summarizes the five areas of the organizational environment with specific examples:

1. Physical environment–physical accessibility
2. Behavior-setting expectations–high vs. low expectations
3. Organizational structure–more or less structured
4. Organizational culture–homogeneity vs. heterogeneity
5. Social climate–control vs. participation

It should be evident that there is some overlap of the above areas. For example, a low-expectation environment of a large, public mental hospital would probably be more highly structured than a smaller agency. A nursing home that has a heterogeneous mix of patients creates a high-expectation environment for the more disabled.

STUDY QUESTIONS

1. You are a direct-service worker employed in a large mental hospital for the severely mentally ill. You are aware that the envi-

ronment of this hospital makes few demands on patients, who spend most of their time watching television. Use the decision-making model to assess the problem and reach a solution.

2. You are the administrator of a community mental health center that serves mentally ill persons discharged from a public mental hospital. You are aware that your staff of psychiatrists, psychologists, nurses, and social workers are not cognizant of the need to take into account the social-ecological environment in the treatment of the service users. What kind of staff recruitment, selection, training, and personnel evaluation program would you develop to remedy this problem?

3. You are a community planner working in the State Office on Aging. The county recently passed a bond issue that provides for construction of halfway houses for the developmentally disabled. You are promulgating an RFP which is to specify the criteria for construction of these facilities. What are some of the criteria and the rationale for their inclusion in the RFP?

4. As a social policy analyst working in the State Department of Health, you have responsibility for writing regulations for health-care facilities, such as general hospitals and nursing homes. A recent survey of patients served by general hospitals indicates that a large proportion are severely disabled. It is your opinion that these hospitals are better equipped to serve acute-illness patients. What kind of regulations would you propose to facilitate a more-appropriate hospital environment for the care of the severely disabled in community general hospitals?

5. As a community planner, you have been given the responsibility to design a comprehensive health-care system for the community, taking into account social-ecological factors. Indicate which social-ecological factors you would take into account in achieving a continuum of care for persons admitted and discharged from institutions.

6. You are a community organizer working with a self-help group for the severely mentally ill. What would you do to assess the organizational climates of the institutions in which members of the group had been previously hospitalized? After you have assembled this data, how would you use it to influence change to achieve service consumer benefit? Indicate the skills you would use.

Chapter 9

ENVIRONMENTAL PRACTICE WITH HIGHLY VULNERABLE POPULATIONS

Environmental Practice with Highly Vulnerable Populations

INTRODUCTION

Vulnerable populations are increasing with the increased prevalence of severe disability as the population ages and medical technologies extend the life of the elderly and newborn. It is estimated that by the year 2000, 65 percent of the population will be 65 years of age or older. The section of the population at greatest risk for severe disability–persons age 85 or older–is growing the fastest (Biegel, Sales, and Schultz 1991). Accompanying this has been a decrease in the availability of a close-knit network of personal care, the result of a loosening of family ties with the shift toward nuclear families and the greater proportion of caretakers who work outside the home (Biegel, Sales, and Schultz 1991; Morris 1977). Reduced fertility rates result in fewer children and siblings to share the burden for future generations of elderly persons (Treas 1981).

Severe disability is linked to chronic illness, which is the number-one health problem in the United States (Anderson and Bauwens 1981:3). Whereas the mortality from infectious diseases declined between 1900 and 1970, the proportions of deaths from major long-term diseases such as heart disease, cancer, and stroke increased more than 250 percent (U.S. Department of Health Education and Welfare 1979). Fifty-two percent of those who seek help in clinics and physicians' offices suffer from long-term illness (Rice and Hodgson 1981). Between two-thirds and three-quarters of the disabled elderly are cared for at home with few or no formal services (Vladeck 1985:9). However, there is evidence that states are increasing economic support for family caregivers of the frail elderly (Biegel et al., 1989). The poor and less-affluent Americans suffer more long-term illness in every age group (Strauss and Corbin 1988:11).

Given the wide prevalence of long-term illness and disability, the role and responsibility of human-service practitioners to serve this group of service consumers becomes increasingly urgent. It is our contention that an environmental focus for practice is most appropriate given the long-term nature of the problem, which limits goals of cure and opens opportunities for enhancing service consumer benefit by creating benevolent environments. Rothman (1994:13-14) advocates environmental interventions for highly vulnerable service users with an emphasis on community-based support in four areas: connecting with community support resources; developing new services; coordinating consumer-centered support systems; and promoting system-wide policy and community education changes.

To illustrate the problems confronting practitioners engaging in environmental practice with the severely disabled, a case situation is presented which will be used throughout this chapter to illustrate how direct service to service users, administration, planning, and policy practice occur in service to the severely disabled. The linkages and interdependencies between micro and macro practice will also be discussed. The six practice skills of decision making, monitoring, leadership, staffing, negotiating, and representing will be illustrated throughout the chapter.

CASE: SEVERE DISABILITY

Mr. D

Mr. D was owner of a small wholesale egg business where, at the age of 70, he fell down an elevator shaft and broke his spinal cord, resulting in loss of control over the lower part of his body. At the time of the accident he was in generally good health, although he suffered from colitis and glaucoma. Treatment at the hospital included intensive physical therapy. After six months of hospital treatment he was discharged to his home, where he lived with his wife. The hospital social worker did not take responsibility to follow up on the social care needs of Mr. D.

A legal suit was instituted against the owner of the building where Mr. D's business was located and the court awarded him $75,000. After this money was exhausted in payment of medical care, workman's compensation insurance assumed responsibility for his medical expenses.

Mrs. D, with her married daughter who lived nearby, had the responsibility for managing the many tasks that needed to be performed to care for Mr. D at home. These included arranging for medical care at home by a general practitioner, and helping him to continue with his physical rehabilitation. Other tasks involved supervising Mr. D's regimen, which eventually enabled him to use a wheelchair; and helping him with his elimination functions, including monitoring the catheter attached to his penis and assisting him in moving his bowels. In order to obtain compensation for medical expenses, the daughter had to assemble receipts and forward them to the insurance company. There was constant need to contact the insurance company to make sure that they paid for the medical expenses. Mr. D's brother, who worked for the insurance company, expedited insurance payments.

Mr. D's disability impacted on the life of the daughter, who was constantly involved in the medical crises of her father and mother. Her full-time job limited her ability to assist her mother with the continual medical crises of her father's illness. However, in times of emergency, she would arrange for transportation to the hospital emergency room. Her social life was affected because of her mother's need for her to be available in case of emergency. The pressures of her parents' problems placed a great strain on her marriage.

Mr. D and his wife supported themselves with income from social security. The wife was confronted with constant pressures to make ends meet. There were frequent medical crises associated with urinary infections resulting in toxemia. Lack of control over his bowels required frequent cleaning of Mr. D and changing of bed linens.

Mrs. D's health suffered under the stress of taking care of her husband. Attempts to obtain a home aide to help with the care of Mr. D were made, but the workman's compensation insurance did not provide for this. The wife suffered from osteoarthritis, which gradually grew worse over the fifteen years she cared for her husband. Mr. D became senile at the age of 84, and began exhibiting violent and uncontrollable behavior. Mrs. D made plans to place him in a nursing home, but at the last minute she "didn't have the heart" to go through with the placement. At the age of 85, Mr. D died at home of a stroke.

Mrs. D

After Mr. D's death, Mrs. D's arthritis worsened. One day her daughter found her lying on the floor, where she had been for several hours. Another time she could not get out of the bathtub. Fortunately, the next-door neighbor heard her shouting and called the daughter. An arrangement was made that elicited the cooperation of the next-door neighbor, who visited Mrs. D regularly to see how she was doing and to help her with food shopping. As Mrs. D became more incapacitated, arrangements were made for a home aide which was paid for through medicaid. Mrs. D found it increasingly difficult to take care of herself and her daughter was concerned that she might start a fire by forgetting to turn off the gas stove.

Mrs. D became more and more depressed after her husband's death. It was evident that taking care of her husband gave her a purpose in life and after he was gone she had nothing to live for. She also developed symptoms of paranoia as a side-effect of the many drugs she was taking. Once these medications were eliminated, the psychological symptoms disappeared.

With her increased physical incapacitation, Mrs. D required more time from a home aide, eventually needing a round-the-clock supervision. As her depression increased, Mrs. D refused to get out of bed despite the urging of the aide. Mrs. D had a very strong personality and throughout her life she played a dominant role in the home and her increasing dependence on others was extremely difficult for her. The aide was not equipped to deal with Mrs. D's strong personality and her refusal to get out of bed. Since this was Mrs. D's home, the aide did not have the authority to influence Mrs. D to do anything she did not want to do. The doctor also was ineffective in changing the situation, since he was focused on Mrs. D's medical needs, rather than her social needs. The lack of physical activity precipitated a minor stroke. She was sent to a local hospital and her psychological condition deteriorated. Her refusal to eat required that she be fed through a tube. Mrs. D complained about the lack of adequate nursing care, as well as the feeling that she was being used a "guinea pig" because of all the tests that she was receiving. After a month, when her health insurance coverage was exhausted, she was placed in a nursing home.

This nursing home required that all patients be out of bed during the day. Mrs. D protested vigorously, but the head nurse was adamant in carrying out this policy. This open expression of anger by Mrs. D resulted in her coming out of her depression and subsequently her adjustment improved. In contrast to her social isolation when she lived in her apartment, Mrs. D interacted regularly with a group of patients who assembled daily. She did this until her death from a stroke two years later.

ISSUES

Acute vs. Severe Disability

Although the creation of positive environments can be beneficial for service consumers who suffer from acute and time-limited problems, it is particularly relevant for persons who require extended care because of long-term problems. The helping professions in general and the health professions in particular have not recognized the need to differentiate services required by persons with acute or severe disabilities (Morrissey and Goldman 1984; Strauss and Glaser 1975). Funding for medical care primarily supports acute-care facilities and only secondarily community-based services (Strauss and Corbin 1988:31). Hospitals do better at meeting the postdischarge needs of acute conditions, but are less effective in linking patients to community-based services equipped to meet long-term needs (Stuen and Monk 1991). Also, since services for the severely disabled are derived from the field of gerontology, they are not appropriate for all persons with long-term illness (Strauss and Corbin 1988:4).

Such social problems as child abuse (Pelton 1981), addiction (Minkoff 1978:29), mental illness (Wintersteen 1986:333), and mental retardation (Dickerson 1981; Wiegerink and Pelosi 1979), as well as problems associated with crime, poverty, and old age, require models of services that have a broader perspective than those developed for persons with acute and time-limited problems. Mechanic (1989) advocates this broader approach for the severely mentally ill, stating that: "manipulating and regulating the context of the illness rather than the illness itself to achieve the best possible outcome given the practical limits of the nature of the condition and the situational contingencies" (201).

The case illustrates the limitations inherent in medical-care system, which neglected Mrs. D's needs for care for her disability. The general hospital could not respond to her psychosocial needs associated with old age. The hospital's stress on diagnostic testing and its inadequate social care reflected the hospital's primary function of treatment of acute medical problems. Although the provision of home care via Medicaid displayed recognition of the importance of physical care in the home it did not provide the kind of social care (e.g., social interaction with peers) that was available in the nursing home.

Impact of Severe Disability on Others

The effect of severe disabilities goes beyond the individual suffering from the problem to include the family (Biegel and Blum 1990). Studies indicate such stresses on family caregivers as: coping with disruptive behaviors associated with cognitive disorders or mental illness; restrictions on social and leisure time activities; infringement of privacy; disruptions of household and work activities; conflicting multiple-role demands (spouse, parent, worker, and caregiver of spouse or in-law); lack of support from other family members; and disruption of family relationships (Biegel, Sales, and Schultz 1991). The negative impact on family caregivers of such long-term illnesses as Alzheimer's disease, cancer, heart disease, and mental illness has been documented (Biegel, Sales, and Schultz 1991).

The movement of deinstitutionalization of the severely disabled has accentuated the need for family care. With regard to the mentally ill, the pressures on families when the patient is in the community are considerable (Morrissey, Tessler, and Farris 1979). The economic, psychological, and social impact of long-term disability on the individual and his/her family requires human service practitioners to develop ongoing support programs for all concerned. For example, a mentally ill or retarded person will require some sort of care for their entire life. Support will also be needed by their families to enable them to constructively aid their disabled relatives. Social support for families of the mentally ill has been found to reduce relapse rates (Falloon, Boyd, and McGill 1984). Interventions for support of family caregivers include group, informational, and direct-service clinical support (Biege, Sales, and Schultz 1991). (See chapters 6 and 7 on social support.)

The stress on family caregivers of the severely disabled is reflected in the many roles performed, including cook, maid janitor, launderer, nursing assistant, transportation provider, mobility supervisor, overseer/administrator of medications, supervisor of special medical equipment, and assistant for personal hygiene, such as toileting and incontinence care, as well as manager of transfers, exercises, feeding, and watching (Lubkin 1986).

The impact of these multiple roles on the family creates paradoxes for the individual as well as the family. Corbin and Strauss (1988) give vivid examples of these dilemmas:

> Coping with the horrors of mutilating surgery and at the same time feeling grateful to be alive; living with the paranoia that arises in response to the vagueness of one's doctors answers when questioned about the future-yet having to trust the doctor because he or she has needed skills; balancing the value of live-in-help against the invasion of privacy; responding to the mate's need for assistance and care yet feeling somewhat resentful that as the caretaker spouse, one can never become tired or ill because there is no one else to take over; willingly using ones's life savings for the medical care of the ill person, while at the same time wondering what lies ahead for one's own future once all that money is gone; wanting to break away from the stress and strain of a relationship torn apart by illness, yet feeling the weight of a legal and moral commitment. (6)

Long-term illness impacts on almost every aspect of life: sex, money, friendship networks, work, the quality of quiet time together, and how relaxed one is (Strauss and Corbin 1988:7).

The case illustrates the great strain on the wife in her caring for her husband. The fact that she was able to do this for 15 years was a testimony of her love for him and her willingness to fulfill her legal and moral commitment to him.

Knowledge and Skill Relevant for Practice with Highly Vulnerable Populations

The knowledge and skill needed to provide services for the severely disabled are of necessity different from that required by persons who have acute problems. The "social side effects" include financial, legal, sexual, marital, and psychological problems as well as a need for assistance with such matters as transportation and household chores (Strauss and Corbin 1988:16). A service strategy that sets realistic goals and persists despite limited gains is essential (Rothman 1994:11). This is evident in hospital social work, where diagnosing, treating, and curing service-consumer problems should be replaced by habilitation techniques directed at functionally restoring persons with long-term disability (Poole 1987:248).

Mechanic's (1989) suggestion that containing disability for the severely mentally ill is preferable to attempting to reverse the condition is applicable to the severely disabled in general.

> Unfortunately, in many areas we lack the necessary knowledge and the technology to do this (cure), and under such conditions it is important to help people cope within the limits of their condition . . . helping individuals live with their conditions are sometimes criticized as defeatist. However, until we have a better understanding of the etiology, course, and treatment of most mental illnesses, it may be more reasonable to attempt to contain disability in this area than to pursue cures without any real knowledge of the ways they are to be achieved. (201)

The severely disabled require an array of supportive services, including housing, socialization, vocational rehabilitation, education, income maintenance, medical care, transportation, homemaker services (Talbott 1981:19). The effectiveness of support is evident in sheltered-care in the community, which predicts better health status compared to care in institutions or in the general community (Segal, Baumohl, and Liése 1993). We know from the accomplishments in the field of physical rehabilitation that much can be accomplished by slow and persistent training of the severely disabled in skills required for daily living. These physical rehabilitation techniques are being transferred to programs for the mentally retarded and mentally ill under the rubric of psychosocial rehabilitation (Anthony, Cohen, and Cohen 1984:137-157; Cnaan et al. 1989; Mechanic 1989:201). The case of Mr. D illustrates how slow and persistent training allowed him to maximize his potential for normalized living in spite of a severe physical handicap.

Effective intervention with severe physical illness requires that medical knowledge be supplemented with a more general approach in order to manage with such problems as social isolation, immobility, social stigmatization, and family disruption (Strauss and Glaser 1975). Current organizational arrangements that emphasize treatment and discharge from institutional care do not provide the aftercare needed to deal with these social side effects and, therefore, are believed to be inadequate and unintentionally "brutal" (Strauss and Corbin 1988:3). Pressure for care of the severely ill in the community has led in recent years to a "home-care boom"–a 242 percent increase in home-care agencies (Dunphy 1984), which are believed to be "poorly organized" (Neifing 1986:306). With the introduction of prospective payment systems in hospitals and the quicker release of patients who are sicker, there are insufficient formal home services to meet greater medical and personal needs (Simon et al. 1995:6). Environmental practice can enhance the effectiveness of hospital discharge planning through better use of home care. This area provides an opportunity for an expanding role for the profession of social work (Cox 1992).

The case illustrates that discharge planning for Mr. D did not adequately provide the family support needed for his care. In the case of Mrs. D, although provision of physical care in the home was generous (e.g., full-time aides), there were some severe limitations in social care. First, the aide was not adequately trained. Second, she did not have the authority to handle a dominant person like Mrs. D, whose refusal to get out of bed precipitated a stroke. The family doctor also was negligent in lack of attention to Mrs. D's social needs. As a result, the social isolation and lack of opportunity for social interaction with peers aggravated her physical and mental condition. Fortunately, this social isolation was remedied in the nursing home. The nursing home provided the authority structure to facilitate the meeting of Mrs. D's social care needs.

DEFINITION

The definition of severe illness is applicable to long-term disability in general. Chronic illness has been defined as "the irreversible presence, accumulation, or latency of disease states or impairments that involve the total human environment for supportive care and self-care, maintenance of function, and prevention of further disability" (Curtin and Lubkin 1986:6). Long-term illnesses: are multiple diseases; are long-term; follow an uncertain course; are disproportionately intrusive upon the individual and their family and are very costly to treat and manage (Strauss and Corbin 1988:11-16).

The severely disabled include a wide variety of groups, including the mentally ill and retarded, the frail elderly, the chemically addicted, the physically ill, the homeless, and child abusers. Institutionalization has been the traditional response to serving the mentally ill and retarded. The neglect and abuse occurring in large congregate institutions has led to deinstitutionalization and widespread discharge into the community. Problems resulting from the lack of provision of community care, in such as homelessness, have stimulated the development of special living arrangements in the community, such as supervised small-group homes.

The *severely mentally ill* include those suffering from psychoses such as schizophrenia and manic depression. The severe nature of this disability results in repeated hospitalizations, because the mentally ill are unable to function in the community. Environmental practice with this group requires ongoing support to facilitate enhancement of their learning, living and working environments (Anthony and Lieberman 1986). Its goal is to provide techniques for changing living situations so that the condition results in the least possible disability (Mechanic 1989:201).

The *developmentally disabled* are another group whose long-term disabilities require environmental interventions. The value of "normalized" environments (Wolfensberger 1972) has been emphasized in the field of mental retardation. Normalization stresses the importance of expectations for normal behavior performance.

The *severely physically ill* include those with such diseases and problems as AIDS; Alzheimer's; cancer; heart disease; arthritis; blindness; deafness; loss of arms and legs; stroke; kidney disease; hypertension; diabetes; congenital anomalies; multiple sclerosis (Schlesinger 1985); and Lyme disease (Logigian, Kaplan, and Steere 1990). The health-care system, with its emphasis on hospital care and the neglect of the social causes and consequences for these illnesses, has influenced the system for caring for the severely ill (Strauss and Corbin

1988). Also, the aging of the population and the attendant disabilities of the frail elderly has had a major impact on the health-care system, including the development of long-term institutional care in nursing homes. The overreliance on hospital care is supported by the Medicare system. A countervailing force is the current emphasis on home care in the proposals for national universal health care, highlighting the relevance of environmentally focused community care.

As indicated, long-term disability of the *frail elderly* has become an increasing problem that requires environmental solutions. Support for the frail elderly comes primarily from their families (Select Committee on Aging 1987). Environmental practice has been directed at providing supportive assistance to enable families to continue their caregiving roles (Biegel and Blum 1990). The case illustrates the absence of professional support to Mr. and Mrs. D in the home.

Chemical addiction (e.g., to drugs and alcohol) is viewed as a cause of long-term disability (Ray and Ksir 1987:346), resulting in child abuse, homelessness, violence, and premature death. "The disease of addiction is chronic, progressive, and degenerative, it is not curable, only arrestible, and one is always prone to relapse" (Manoleas 1992:125). Addiction is seen as rooted in social life-style requiring ongoing and continuous environmental support as provided in self-help groups like Alcoholics Anonymous and Narcotic Anonymous. Influencing the environment is an important means of affecting patients' attitudes toward alcohol rehabilitation (Mechanic 1961).

The case illustrates two kinds of severe disability. Mr. D's disability resulted from an accident. It was fortunate that he was covered by workers' compensation insurance, which provided for long-term medical care in the home. However, this coverage did not include nursing and social care, resulting in the overburdening of Mrs. D and worsening her disability from old age. However, she was fortunate in that she lived in a state that provided extensive home care financed by Medicaid.

INTERVENTIONS

Trajectory Model of Long-Term Illness

Strauss and Corbin's (1988) "trajectory" model indicates what is involved in the management of incurable illnesses. Although this model was developed for the care of the severely physically ill, it provides a socially based framework that can be applied to environmental interventions for long-term disability in general. This model will be described, followed by a discussion of its implications for environmental practice in direct service, administration, community organizing, planning, and policymaking.

This model emphasizes the active role that professionals, the disabled, the family, and whoever else is involved take in the *social management* of the course of the illness. It assumes that there are work tasks that need to be accomplished in the day-to-day management of the illness in addition to such responsibilities as housekeeping, child rearing, and earning a living. In the case, the responsibility for managing the care of Mr. D fell primarily to his wife, since the daughter's role was limited by her having a full-time job.

The management tasks require an environmental focus on controlling and shaping the course of the disability. In the case, Mrs. D had to carry out a multitude of tasks to care for her husband at home. The daughter also had to constantly apply pressure to obtain coverage by the insurance company. Except for the help of the doctor, who was primarily concerned with physical care, they performed these tasks without much assistance from professionals.

Persistent professional effort is required of the environmental practitioner to counter the sense of hopelessness that comes over acute-care professionals because of the slowness of recovery of these service users. This was evident in the case, where the acute-care hospital, with its goal of cure, placed patients in a passive role with low behavior expectations. In contrast, the nursing home was better able to serve Mrs. D because they had a structure which stressed high behavior expectations.

The lack of integrated and coordinated service-delivery systems– (White 1987:96) calls it a "nonsystem"–has particular impact on the severely disabled, with the result that they often fall between institutional cracks in the system. This requires a role for the environmental practitioner to manipulate the system to insure that the these disabled will receive the care they need (Strauss and Corbin 1988:66-68). This is illustrated in the case where the lack of coordination of medications received by Mrs. D resulted in severe side effects.

Intrinsic to this task of responding to the reality of severe disability is the need for the environmental practitioner to appreciate that the professional view is constrained by an inevitable piecemeal approach, coming as it is from the standpoint of particular specialties, professional positions and ideologies (Neugeboren 1991; Strauss and Corbin 1988:42). This can be countered somewhat by encouraging feedback from the service users and their families. The environmental practitioner should act as a communication link between service consumers and their families and service providers, facilitating feedback to inform the latter on what interventions are more or less effective.

In the case, the lack of coordination of the medication received by Mrs. D could have been obviated if an environmental practitioner was available to act as a link between the patient and the several physicians who were prescribing these medications.

Intervention Areas

The trajectory model for chronic illness includes the following areas for intervention: (1) illness phases; (2) management of the illness; (3) resources needed; (4) arrangements; (5) biographical work; and (6) articulation.

Illness Phases

Illness phases are the components of the life cycle of long-term illness: diagnosis, acute, recovery, stable, unstable, deteriorating, and dying. The management of these phases, most of which take place at home, provides a context for environmental practice, with the major concern of the disabled and their families being the maintenance of quality of life despite the limitations in functioning. Environmental practice with the long-term disabled is shaped by the fact that long-term illness requires lifelong work to control its course, manage its symptoms, and live with the resulting disability. The environmental practitioner's interventions will depend on the trajectory phase and the work required to manage the disability in that illness stage. Thus, the acute phase requires activities linked to intensive work to stabilize the service user, in contrast to the stable phase, where less intensive monitoring is needed.

The different stages of long-term illness are illustrated in the case. For Mr. D, the first acute phase was in the hospital after the accident. Here, professional assistance focused on acute medical care. Supportive care for the family was not available to help plan for his return home.

The extended nature of the care needed by the long-term disabled is usually managed by family members. For those who lack family support and direction, there is a real danger of the person not receiving care to facilitate maximum functioning, resulting in custodial care in institutions (Strauss and Corbin 1988:67). The case illustrates how Mrs. D was able to care for her husband until his death without having to resort to institutionalization. In contrast, the opposite was the case for Mrs. D, who had to be placed in a nursing home because there was no one to care for her at home. At that point, Mrs. D could have been cared for at home since she had suffered only a minor stroke. However, the daughter made the decision to have her placed because she was overwhelmed by the responsibility of dealing with the many medical emergencies. An environmental practitioner in this situation could have provided the determination and support to motivate the daughter to persist in home care despite the relapses.

Each phase involves different processes. The *diagnostic* phase involves a quest for an understanding of the cause of symptoms. This may involve a fairly rapid identification of cause leading to an easy diagnosis. Other situations can entail a lengthy search with unreliable tests (false positives and negatives) and delayed diagnosis. The environmental practitioner's task is to help the service user to obtain information on the competence of the diagnosticians and to facilitate getting second opinions. When the evaluation is uncertain and the patient is placed in "diagnostic limbo" (Corbin and Strauss 1988:28), the environmental practitioner will need to provide the support needed to enable the service consumer to pursue the quest to a successful conclusion. In the case situation, the family was concerned about the paranoid symptoms, which initially were diagnosed as mental illness. Later, it was discovered that these symptoms were the result of negative drug interactions. Inappropriate treatment also occurred when Mrs. D was treated for depression after she was hospitalized. The symptoms were alleviated after she was placed in the more appropriate environment of a nursing home.

The *acute* phase requires intensive intervention, usually in an institutional setting. The environmental practitioner collaborates with hospital staff in facilitating discharge and plans for community care. In the case, Mrs. D carried the full burden of the care of her husband. The hospital social worker did not provide the necessary assistance to enable Mrs. D to obtain nursing and social care in the home to help her with the care of her husband.

The *recovery* phase involves three processes: "mending," or the healing process; "stretching capacities," (i.e., pushing the person to the boundaries of his/her current abilities); and "reknitting," (i.e., putting the ill person back together within the actual and perceived limitations of body and social performance) (Strauss and Corbin 1988:59-60). In the case, Mr. D's physical rehabilitation therapy in the hospital enabled him to be discharged to his home. This therapy continued in the home, enabling him to get out of bed and into a wheelchair. Given his severe physical limitations, Mr. D functioned well and to the surprise of the professionals survived for 15 years.

The environmental practitioner needs to insure that family and other professionals do not err on the side of setting expectations too low, thus reinforcing the sick role for the disabled and reducing the potential for recovery. In the case, Mrs. D's deterioration after her husband's death was exacerbated by inappropriately low expectations of her, in that she was allowed to stay in bed which precipitated a stroke.

The *stable* phase requires the integration of stabilizing regimens and disability with the ongoing patterns of life. A major contributor to stabilization is a cooperative spouse or other intimate caretaker. Contributing conditions are adequate financing, housing, accommodating employers and work colleagues, counseling services and physical therapy (Strauss and Corbin 1988:97). Environmental practice facilitates the coordination of the above resources. In the case, Mr. D's condition was stabilized for a number of years, primarily because of his spouse, in contrast to Mrs. S, who deteriorated in the absence of an intimate caretaker.

It is in the stable phase that information on the uniqueness of the service users' reactions to various conditions such as drugs, types of activities and environmental conditions should be collected and communicated to service providers and significant others to prevent relapse. It is during this stage that persons assume the role of *agents*. Controlling agents monitor the use of medication. Protecting agents act in emergency situations, such as with epileptics who have a severe seizures. In the case, the wife and daughter were the principal agents who monitored the medication and acted in emergency situations, as when Mr. D developed toxemia because of a malfunction of the catheter. In Mrs. D's case, the daughter served this agent function.

The *unstable* phase for the long-term disabled is related to the fluctuations in service consumer functioning. Such physical illnesses as arthritis, migraine, allergies, and asthma, as well as such mental conditions as schizophrenia and depression, have their ups and downs. In contrast to the acute phase, where there is motivation to stabilize the service consumer, the unstable phase challenges the support system's patience to persevere. This is important, since lapses may be temporary, with the professionals being unable to determine the cause. Service consumers in this phase may in desperation turn to drastic alternative forms of service such as severe diet regimes, which require life-style changes.

In the case, the constant fluctuations in Mr. D's function were a severe challenge to Mrs. D and the daughter. Their perseverance enabled Mr. D. to survive for many years.

Instability may also be induced by iatrogenic treatments such as negative reactions to medication. One in four persons over 65 years of age are given prescriptions that have negative side effects (Kolata 1994). Negative drug interactions are not uncommon for persons receiving uncoordinated treatment for multiple illnesses. This is the case often for the elderly (Mechanic 1978:348; Illich 1976; Bosk 1979; Spitzer 1980). Cumulative negative effects of medications are linked to long-term use and requires detoxification services (Strauss and Corbin 1988:108). In the case, Mrs. D's development of paranoid symptoms was a direct result of negative drug interactions.

The *deterioration* phase includes early, middle, and late stages. In the early stage, the individual needs aid to come to terms with their disability and concern over future problems. In the middle stage the person may have to cut back on responsibilities such as a job, driving a car, or housekeeping work. In the later stage of deterioration, the individual can benefit from home-care services. During these stages, social arrangements need to be adjusted according to the requirements of the particular stage. Changes in resources, such as unavailability of the caretaker through divorce, death of spouse, or marriage of a child, can affect the social arrangements.

Management of the Illness

Each of the above phases require different management responsibilities that necessitate following a regimen within the context of everyday life, in which such work as housekeeping, child rearing, and earning a living must go on. Management responsibilities includes carrying out different tasks: who does them, how they vary in degree of difficulty and amount of time it takes to complete them in relation to the phase of the illness. These tasks include: controlling symptoms; monitoring, preventing, and managing crises; carrying out regimens; managing limitations of activity; stretching the limitations of activity; and preventing or living with social isolation. It also involves "contextualizing the illness into one's biography," (i.e., making it part of ongoing life by coming to terms with the illness itself, the limitations it imposes, and the possibility of death, and restructuring new conceptions of the self in light of the illness and the bodily changes it brings) (Corbin and Strauss 1988:10). Other types of tasks include: obtaining and maintaining a paid position; maintaining a marriage; running and keeping up a home; and raising a child. Management responsibilities intrude on the life of those surrounding the patient, including family, caretakers, friends, neighbors, and professionals. The environmental practitioner needs to be aware of these management responsibilities in order to help access the formal resources needed to accomplish and coordinate these management tasks.

In the case, the severe disabilities of Mr. and Mrs. D impacted on the life of the daughter, whose social life was constrained by the demands for her to be available to assist with medical emergencies, first with her father and then with her mother. This had a major impact on her marriage.

Patients and their families necessarily develop knowledge and skill in the management of long-term disability. Learning from their day-to-day experiences, they develop the ability to monitor and evaluate professional competencies to provide safe care with regard to medication, as well as other aspects of service (Strauss et al. 1985). Professional training of patients and their families in the management of illness is desirable, but is often neglected due to the overemphasis on acute care (Guillemin and Holstrom 1986). This requires a variety of "resources."

Resources Needed

The kind and amount of resources needed also will vary with phases of the illness. Such resources as family and friends, knowledge of how to obtain competent care, and financial aid may have to be sought out, bargained for, or purchased. Resources adequate for one phase may be insufficient for another one.

Information is an important resource, especially with regard to the availability and appropriateness of formal services. Since long-term disability by definition suggests lack of success in remediation of the problem, there may be the possibility that the service being provided is not appropriate. In the field of health care, there is increasing evidence that traditional medical solutions need to be supplemented by complementary systems of intervention. Examples of complementary care would include nutrition for treatment of heart disease, arthritis, cancer, etc. (Atkins 1988; Fredericks 1981); yoga to reduce high blood pressure; chiropractic for muscular skeletal problems; and acupuncture for drug abuse (Smith 1988).

Useful information includes knowledge of which services are more or less effective for different kinds of disabilities. For example, psychotherapy is contraindicated for the severely mentally ill, in contrast to educational approaches used in teaching skills for everyday living (Rubin 1985). Self-help groups of patients and families are an important evaluative source where information is shared as to which helping sources are most effective (Whittaker et al. 1983). Effective management of resources also requires a variety of "arrangements."

As indicated previously, interventions to support family caregivers have been categorized as group, education, and clinical support. Support-group interventions provide caretakers with emotional support, informational support, and enhancement of coping skills. Support groups are either professionally led and time limited, or peer led, usually of an ongoing nature. Educational interventions include the professional provision of information and/or skills to enable the care-givers to function more effectively. Cognitive and skill development includes: cognitive information, self-enhancement skills, and behavioral management skills. Clinical or direct-service interventions involve a variety of treatment services, including: counseling/therapy, respite, behavioral/cognitive stimulation, hospice, day hospital, and general psychosocial interventions (Biegel, Sales, and Schultz 1991).

The unpredictability of the course of severe disability requires constant balancing of resource allocation between demands of daily life and the needs of the service consumer. Priorities need to be continually set in order to determine where time, money, and effort should be directed. The environmental practitioner aids the service user and the family in establishing and implementing these priorities. Maintaining this equilibrium requires activity that has been termed "management in process," which emphasizes adaptation to change. Management in process includes the following work process: (1) calculating and allocating resources; (2) maintaining a division of labor; (3) planning and coordinating the total work; and (4) sustaining the motivation and commitment of the service consumer and family (Corbin and Strauss 1988:118). The environmental practitioner needs to assess "the competition among lines of work, unbalanced workloads, conditions that tend to disrupt the established routines, and the factors upon which motivation to continue work is contingent" (Corbin and Strauss 1988:125).

In the case Mrs. D had to calculate and allocate the funds obtained from social security and workman's compensation. A division of labor was established in which the daughter dealt with the insurance company while the mother took care of her husband. The motivation and commitment of the daughter was not sustained, resulting in the placement of Mrs. D in a nursing home.

Arrangements

Environmental arrangements are developed within the context of the home and family life and work activities and schedules. Most arrangements involve organizing the time and tasks of the disabled in conjunction with those of family members, and sometimes those of relatives, friends, and neighbors. These arrangements involve different kinds of *agents,* such as rescuing agent, protective agents, assisting agents, or control agents (Strauss et al. 1984:17). In the case, arrangements were made with the next-door neighbor, who served as a protective agent for Mrs. D in times of emergency, as well as an assisting agent who helped with food shopping. The daughter served as a rescuing agent for both parents. Life contingencies force rearrangements and require continuous efforts (Strauss and Corbin 1988:48). A major focus is the linking of efforts of formal and informal care systems (Neugeboren 1990). In the case, Mr. D's brother was a link between the family and the insurance company who helped to facilitate payment of medical expenses.

Biographical Work

Biographical work deals with the destructive psychological impact that severe disability has on those who are disabled, their friends, and their families. To some, long-term disability becomes the main focus of daily life. However, others are able to integrate the illness so that it does not completely dominate and exclude other aspects of living (Corbin and Strauss 1988). The strains of prolonged disability result in changes in household arrangements, job situations, and social relationships. Biographical work by the environmental practitioner assists in dealing with problems of identity and finding new goals in life or new ways of achieving old ones. It requires the establishment of some social distancing to protect those impacted by the long-term illness from being overwhelmed by the never-ending pressures and burdens associated with the management of long-term disability (Beattie 1987). In the case, the burdens of care, first for Mr. D and then for Mrs. D, pretty much overwhelmed all family members. Employment of the daughter enabled her to obtain some social distance from the pressures generated by the severe disabilities of her mother and father.

Articulation

Coordinating of all the arrangements, resources, agents, and tasks requires articulation skills. Keeping all of the constituents together is difficult, given unexpected contingencies of living. Intrinsic to articulation is the use of negotiating skills in the coordination of the various agents and tasks.

Now that we have concluded discussion of the trajectory model, we will proceed to apply this framework to environmental micro and macro practice in the organizational, community, and societal arenas.

Organizational Arena

Direct Service

Intervention on the direct-service level would be influenced by *illness phases*. The *acute* phase, which often takes place in an institutional setting, requires the direct-service worker to work intensively, given the pressures for discharge to the community. This direct-service work will require collaborative efforts, utilizing negotiating skills with other hospital staff and community agencies in planning for discharge.

Direct practice in other phases, such as the recovery, stable, unstable, deteriorated, and dying stages, takes place for the most part in the home. As the disability progresses and the need for resources increases, the direct practitioner can be instrumental in informing service users of the availability of these resources. Resources for long-term care may be more available to the poor through such programs as Medicaid. For the middle class, who are ineligible for long-term care through funded means-based programs, it may be necessary for a skilled resource coordinator (see Chapter 4) to use negotiation skills to link them to aid for which they are eligible.

A case-management service for the middle-class frail elderly has been developed using a private practice model. The National Association of Professional Geriatric Care Managers (NAPGCM) is an alliance of private practice professionals. This organization publishes a newsletter, standards for practice, a national directory, and a code of ethics (NAPGCM 1993). This service-delivery approach has particular relevance for an advocacy stance for the disabled since there are fewer organizational constraints on the practitioner in this model. This linkage includes the coordination of formal and informal care.

The above role of the direct-service practitioner will require negotiating skills. Whether the task is discharge planning from a hospital setting or doing resource coordination, the direct-service person will need to determine whether and how professionals and organizations are interdependent and where there is potential for a resource exchange derived from shared goals.

A key to illness management is understanding the impact of the context of everyday living on the different phases of the illness. "Contextualizing the illness" (Corbin and Strauss 1988:2) requires activities that respond to the changing relationships and resource requirements as the individual moves through different stages of the disability. Intrinsic to a broad view of the illness course is understanding the concept of continuity of care. The influence of lifestyles must be integrated with illness management to insure that the patient and the family will follow through on the arrangements needed to integrate the illness and their everyday life.

The direct-service environmental practitioner needs to understand more than psychological and psychiatric concepts such as coping and stress. The practitioner needs to discover for each service consumer "the meaning of his or her body–its images, appearances, perceived limitations, failures and successes in performance-and above all the body's relations to one's sense of self" (Corbin and Strauss 1988:67).

Administration

The function of administration of programs for the long-term disabled is to insure service effectiveness by formulating appropriate organizational goals, designing agency structures relevant to these objectives, and implementing programs to accomplish these aims.

Formulation of Goals. The formulation of environmentally oriented goals to serve the severely disabled emphasizes social care goals. This accomplishment is the task of upper-level institutional leadership (see Chapter 2). Other responsibilities of executive leadership are: legitimating the organization; selecting service technologies; developing internal structures; and initiating change (Selznick 1957).

As indicated previously, the formulation of environmentally relevant goals requires the administrator to obtain support and sanction from funding authorities, governing boards, and staff. This will help legitimate the new organizational mission. Staff and community resistance can be expected when agency goals are changed to serve the severely disabled, requiring strategies to overcome this opposition.

This can be illustrated in the case, where the rehabilitation goals of the hospital in which Mrs. D was hospitalized were not appropriate for the severely disabled. If this hospital decided to add social-care goals it might anticipate much resistance from the medical community, who are committed to practice with the acutely ill. However, given the prevalence of long-term illness, it would seem probable that support could be marshaled to overcome this opposition. A strategy that some hospitals have used to meet the needs of the severely disabled elderly is to build or purchase long-term care facilities.

Design of Organizational Structures. The selection of organizational structures appropriate for serving the long-term disabled includes the design of service technologies (*role structure*) pertinent for caring for this population group. In the case of a community hospital, the roles of physicians, nurses, social workers, and others would need to stress knowledge and skill in the environmental practice area.

The design of *authority structures* to provide the sanctions to facilitate the accomplishment of social-care goals is also required. In the above example of a hospital moving toward these goals, physicians, nurses and other staff who have the expertise in environmental practice would be given positions of authority to ensure the implementation of these social-care goals. For example, doctors and nurses educated in public health would be placed in these positions. Social workers educated in community practice would also be appropriate.

Since interagency relations are a basic part of environmental practice for the disabled, the *interorganizational structure* would also need to be changed. Administrators could accomplish this by selecting community agencies in their "organizational set" and planning for the development of affiliation agreements to facilitate patient referrals. In the case of an acute-care hospital, affiliation agreements with nursing homes and public health nursing agencies would allow for better service to the severely disabled.

Community Arena

Social Advocacy and Community Organization

Social advocacy interventions mobilize and represent the interests and needs of the severely disabled. Community organizers communicate to administrators, planners, and policymakers information obtained from service user groups on the adequacy and effectiveness of the services they receive. Citizen advocacy agencies represent the interests of the disabled by writing position papers based on systematic study. They publicize these reports via the media and by sharing them with policymakers. Public demonstrations are a strategy used by social advocates to publicize the needs of the disabled.

In the case of the community hospital, social advocates direct their influence toward health-planning councils, whose approval is needed for hospital construction. They can persuade community health-planning boards to include architectural standards that promote normalized environments in hospitals as part of the criteria for grant approval.

Planning

Community planning agencies play an important role in influencing service provision for the long-term disabled. Their funding of these programs places them in a key position to monitor and coordinate services for the severely disabled. Poor linkage between institutional and community care agencies is a major barrier to effective service to the long-term disabled. Community planners have a responsibility to facilitate better coordination between these two service sectors.

Another planning need is an integration of medical and social services that takes into account the interdependencies of these two areas of need (Strauss and Corbin 1988:126). The case illustrates this need with respect to the hospital and the physicians in private practice. The integration of medical and social services will require the use of decision-making and negotiating skills. Decision-making skills would be used to define the problem and evaluate alternative solutions to achieve this integration. Overcoming the lack of coordination between institutional and community-care agencies will also require negotiating skills.

Societal Arena

Policy Formulation

Policy-formulating agencies such as legislative committees have the responsibility of examining current policies to determine how they impact on service to the severely disabled. Policy analysts use a framework (see Chapter 2) in which policy change is viewed in terms of change in substantive goals and/or procedures to achieve these goals. Decision-making skills are used to formulate problems and evaluate alternative solutions in order to develop more appropriate goals and the strategies for achieving the goal of service to the long-term disabled.

Change in Substantive Goals. Goal clarification is the process of assessing the relationship of means and ends of human service programs. It helps to avoid goal displacement, whereby service user benefit becomes secondary to the methods used to achieve this goal. Application of goal clarification to policies on financing long-term community care for the disabled would reveal that although there are some provisions for financial assistance for particular groups, such as veterans, persons on welfare, and some of the physically disabled (e.g., spinal cord injuries), there is inadequate provision for in-home care on a long-term basis for the severely ill and disabled in general and more specifically for the middle-class (Strauss and Corbin 1988:118). This is important because there is evidence that there is a 40 percent savings from home care compared with nursing-home care (Cheung 1988). The policy practitioner needs to formulate new funding policies to redress the imbalance in financing for long-term care. Decision-making skills are needed to analyze the problem, including the role that various provider groups have played.

Shift in Goal Priorities. A shift in goal priorities would address the current imbalance which gives preference to acute short-term care and neglects long-term care for the severely disabled. Decision-making skills would be used to understand the forces that have resulted in the priority given to short-term care. Problem formulation would analyze the influence of acute-care organizations (e.g., general hospitals) on this imbalance and seek solutions that take into account the pressures on these agencies for service to the severely disabled.

Change in Strategies for Achieving Goals. In the formulation of policy for service to the severely disabled, changes in strategies for achieving goals may need to be considered. One strategy for achieving goals is related to the way an organization deals with its environment, e.g., by using closed- or open-system approaches. Closed-system strategies assume that human service agencies can be independent, and do not need the aid of other organizations. An open-system strategy assumes interdependence between human service organizations. As indicated in the situation of community hospitals, there have been efforts to develop comprehensive human service centers, including the provision of long-term care. This is an example of a closed-system strategy.

One can question whether this a viable strategy, given the multitude of needs of the severely disabled. An open-system approach may be more suitable; however this requires active efforts to establish linkages with other community agencies.

INTEGRATION OF MICRO AND MACRO ENVIRONMENTAL PRACTICE

The integration of micro and macro environmental practice in service to the long-term disabled will require the linking of administrative and the direct service functions. This is accomplished by the use of monitoring, coordinating, and staffing skills.

Monitoring

Monitoring of service delivery is a critical administrative function given the problems of discontinuity in coordination and integration of services for the long-term disabled. Tracking of service delivery can reveal gaps in provision and minimize the problem of service consumers falling between the cracks in the service system (Rothman 1994:189-190). Intrinsic to effective monitoring is a system of ongoing and continuous evaluative feedback from service users and their families. Communication between direct-service staff and administration is critical for the determination of service gaps. This can be done through systematic assessment of unmet needs in open and closed cases. This would require administrative and direct-service staff to have monitoring skills.

In the case, the hospital neglected to monitor the deleterious effects of the lack of social-care services for Mrs. D, resulting in the deepening of her depression and her refusal to eat.

Coordinating

Lack of cooperative working relationships between service agencies has major negative consequences for the severely disabled in view of their multiplicity of needs. The role of administration in promoting better coordination between agencies is critical. Coordination is also important between formal and informal (e.g., family) care systems (Brody 1981; Neugeboren 1990; Rothman 1994; Vladeck 1983). Formal coordination between service agencies is accomplished by affiliation agreements.

In the case situation, there was a lack of coordination between the various medical specialists in prescribing medication for Mrs. D, resulting in a negative interaction that caused psychotic symptoms. If this were to occur in a case in an agency, it would be the responsibility of administration to establish communication structures for coordinating information between providers to avoid this kind of problem. One mechanism that could be used is a computer program that allows the pharmacist to check for drug interaction.

This task of coordination would require that staff have the ability (i.e., negotiating, skills) to determine the extent to which resource (e.g., information) exchange is possible based on the extent that the different parties have shared goals.

Staffing

Staff recruitment and selection policies would need to focus on obtaining personnel with the philosophy and skills appropriate for environmental practice with the long-term disabled. In-service training would be needed to reeducate existing staff who do not have these skills. Personnel performance-evaluation systems should also be formulated to ensure that staff are functioning appropriately in their service to the severely disabled. A university-based training program for serving the long-term mentally ill has provided in-service training for staff in agencies providing these services (Anthony, Cohen, and Cohen 1984). Teachers of preventive medicine have given particular attention to preparing physicians for practice with the long-term disabled (Clark and Williams 1976).

In the case, the hospital should have had staff recruitment and selection policies to insure that personnel had the environmentally oriented skills needed to serve the long-term disabled. Staff in-service training would also help the staff to understand the social needs of the frail elderly, particularly in the area of discharge planning. This would require the use of staffing skills in the human resources department of the hospital.

SUMMARY

This chapter has reviewed the policy and practice issues in environmental practice for the long-term disabled. The trajectory model for the care of the severely ill was presented as an environmentally focused framework for service to the long-term disabled. Implications of this model for direct service, administration, planning, social advocacy and social policy practice was also discussed. A case was used throughout the chapter to illustrate how the concepts and intervention skills can be applied to practice.

STUDY QUESTIONS

1. You are a direct-service social worker employed in the nursing home where Mrs. D was placed. What are some of the interventions you would plan to help Mrs. D and her daughter? What are the skills that you would need to accomplish these interventions?

2. You are the administrator of the hospital where Mr. D was placed. Indicate some of the steps you would take to ensure that more effective discharge planning would occur in situations similar to that of Mr. D. What skills would you use to accomplish the above?

3. You are a community planner. What activities would you engage in to ensure better coordination between hospitals and nursing homes in the care of the severely disabled? Indicate how these activities would affect the D family. Indicate the skills you would use.

4. You are a community organizer working in a social advocacy agency. Develop an advocacy program to address the lack of social-care services for the severely disabled at the local community hospital.

5. You are policy analyst working for the legislature in the state where the D family resides. What kind of legislative policies would you formulate to help deal with the problems confronted by the D family? What skills would you use?

6. You are the administrator of the hospital where Mrs. D was placed. Indicate what kind of policy changes you would make to ensure that the frail elderly would receive more appropriate care at the hospital. Discuss the skills you would need to accomplish the above.

Chapter 10

ENVIRONMENTAL PRACTICE IMPLICATIONS

Environmental Practice Implications

I. Intervention Skills
    A. Implications for Service Delivery
    B. Implications for Education and Training
    C. Implications for Research
II. Resource Coordination
    A. Implications for Service Delivery
    B. Implications for Education and Training
    C. Implications for Research
III. Social Support
    A. Implications for Service Delivery
    B. Implications for Education and Training
    C. Implications for Research
IV. Organizational Environments
    A. Implications for Service Delivery
    B. Implications for Education and Training
    C. Implications for Research
V. Practice with Vulnerable Populations
    A. Implications for Service Delivery
    B. Implications for Education and Training
    C. Implication for Research
VI. Implications for Other Areas of Environmental Practice
VII. Integration of Micro and Macro Practice
    A. Implications for Service Delivery
    B. Implications for Education and Training
    C. Implications for Research
VIII. Conclusions

This concluding chapter discusses the implications of the five broad environmental practice areas (intervention skills, resource coordination, social support, organizational environments, and service to vulnerable populations) for service delivery, education, training, and research in the human services. Implications for the integration of micro and macro practice, as well as for other environmental practice areas, will also be discussed.

INTERVENTION SKILLS

Implications for Service Delivery

The six intervention skills (decision making, leadership, monitoring, representing, staffing, and negotiating) present a multidimensional approach to service interventions by showing how they occur in different arenas of practice, their technical aspects, and structural contexts. This has implications for practice, which traditionally has been defined unidimensionally, stressing primarily individual practitioner competencies. Viewing practice skills as a complex configuration of individual technical capacities in interaction with situational contingencies presents a challenge in the design of service-delivery systems. Agencies committed to environmental change will need to reformulate the roles of practitioners as well as the supporting structures that take into account this multidimensional definition of intervention skills.

Implications for Education and Training

The multidimensional delineation of environmental intervention skills has special implications for education and training. In-service training programs in organizations adopting the mission of environmental change will face the substantial task of retraining staff who for the most part are products of person-changing education programs.

Formal professional-education programs in schools of social work, psychology, medicine, nursing, and other human service fields will also have to modify their curricula and recruit teaching personnel who can instruct students in environmental intervention skills. Since the literature and textbooks on environmental practice have yet to be written, faculty and students will have to learn from those engaged in this kind of practice. Field internship programs can be used as a vehicle to accomplish this objective.

Implications for Research

The further development of environmental intervention skills will require systematic research on the effectiveness of this multidimensional model of practice skills. Studies of actual practice may reveal that skills other than those discussed here will have to be included as part of an array of intervention methods (e.g., legal and political skills). It also would be useful to study the relationship between the technical and situational components between environmental practice skills in terms of achieving service consumer benefit.

RESOURCE COORDINATION

Implications for Service Delivery

The acceptance of community resource coordination as a basic component of environmental practice can have significant implications for the design of human service programs. The coordination aspect of case management and discharge planning is becoming an increasingly important component in service-delivery systems, not only in the public and nonprofit agencies, but also in managed care (Kane 1992) in the for-profit human service sector (e.g., health care). Resource coordination, which requires knowledge and skill in interorganizational practice, will necessitate the modification of agency structures on all levels in order to implement community resource-coordination objectives. New roles for direct-service workers, as well as for administrators, planners, and policy analysts, will need to be formulated and sanctioned. Caseworkers will need to use social-exchange strategies to obtain resources for service users from other agencies. Administrators will need to develop the organizational skills to achieve the interagency collaboration that is the foundation of community resource coordination. Resource data banks will need to be established on the agency, community, and state levels as a necessary support for community resource coordination.

Implications for Education and Training

Implementation of community resource coordination as a component of environmental practice has substantial implications for in-service training programs of agencies moving in this direction. Training will be required for *all* staff to ensure that they have the knowledge and skill to carry out the necessary tasks involved in community resource coordination. Focus will have to be on the importance of concrete resources, where they are located in the community, and how to overcome barriers and gain access to them.

The curricula of professional schools will need to incorporate content on community resource coordination on both the micro and macro levels. Theories of social exchange, which is the foundation of service coordination, will need to be included in courses in case management, discharge planning, and management.

Implications for Research

Although there has been some useful research on coordination, with a focus on the process (Aiken et al. 1975), there is a need to examine the collaborative relations between micro and macro practitioners to achieve effective community resource coordination. A question that could be posed for systematic study is what kinds of structural supports are effective in facilitating successful resource coordination on the direct-service level?

SOCIAL SUPPORT

Implications for Service Delivery

Social support as key aspect of environmental practice has implications for the design of service-delivery systems. The inclusion of systems of formal and informal care as an integral part of service delivery will require modifications of organizational structures and philosophies to facilitate collaboration between the two different systems. This has implications for equality between the professionals in the formal care systems and the nonprofessional lay persons who make up the informal care systems. Formal organizations will need to develop new structures to promote equality to prevent the domination of the informal community networks by the professionals and to ensure the usefulness of mutual aid and self-help for service users.

Implications for Education and Training

The promotion of social support as an integral component of human service will require modification of in-service training programs. Members of the lay community-support systems could be included as teaching aides for in-service training classes in order to help staff gain an appreciation of their potential roles in assisting them and the service consumers.

Professional education will also have to be modified to include participation of lay persons in educational programs. Students can gain an understanding of the value of social support by participating in self-help groups through field internships.

Implications for Research

Evaluation of social support interventions could focus on the relationship between lay citizens and professionals in the delivery of human services. Another area for research is the extent to which social support can achieve prevention objectives.

ORGANIZATIONAL ENVIRONMENTS

Implications for Service Delivery

Environmental practice that takes into account organizational environments can have significant implications for service-delivery systems. In contrast with the traditional emphasis solely on the problems of the service consumer, an organizationally focused intervention would emphasize the ways in which the organization impacts on the person. Information systems for assessing agency environments would need to be developed in order to intermesh the needs of the individual and the agency environment.

Implications for Education and Training

The task of in-service training will be to provide staff with an understanding of the opportunities and constraints that organizational environments impose on the referral process. Agency personnel, in deciding what types of service user should be referred to which kind of agency, will need to be trained to understand how the individual service consumer's needs are affected by different types of organizational environments.

Professional education will have to give greater recognition to the fact that human services are agency-based, requiring that curricula include content on organizational knowledge and skill. Knowledge of how the organization impacts on practice and the skills to cope with these influences should be the foundation of education in the human services. The accrediting body in social work education has recently recognized the importance of this knowledge (Curriculum Policy Statement 1992), although in the past the Human Behavior and Social Environment curriculum component has tended to neglect this content area (Neugeboren 1994).

Implications for Research

Research on how organizational environments impact on individual service user's needs would be useful in guiding practitioners' case-referral decisions enabling a better fit between consumer and agency. A study of the impact of centralized vs. decentralized agency structures on various types of service consumers could also be an aid to organizational design.

PRACTICE WITH VULNERABLE POPULATIONS

Implications for Service Delivery

An environmentally oriented model for service to highly vulnerable populations has implications for a service-delivery system for this consumer group. The application of the trajectory service-delivery model to disabled groups who require long-term care–such as the mentally ill, developmentally disabled, severely physically ill, and the frail elderly–will require service-delivery structures different from those presently used for service to persons with acute short-term difficulties. These structures will need to focus on the relationships between institutional and community care with resources shifted from the former to the latter form of care.

Implications for Education and Training

The environmental approach to service for highly vulnerable populations will require a retooling of human service personnel. In-service training will have to focus on developing a different service philosophy that combines both high expectations for the active participation of service consumers, as well as has a commitment to slow and gradual progress over an extended time period.

Professional education will also have to modify the philosophy underlying practice with this population group, as well the specific intervention skills. Again, education will need to rely on the knowledge and skill available in programs that currently service this population group through the use of field practicums. An effort in this direction is the collaboration between California's schools of social work and county social service departments for training in the public social services (Specht and Courtney 1994:150), an arena that includes service to vulnerable populations (Neugeboren 1970a). The building of a community-based system of social care will require funding from the national government (Specht and Courtney 1994:172)

Implications for Research

Research will be needed to evaluate the utility of the trajectory intervention model for service to groups other than the severely physically ill for whom it was developed. Will the different stages and tasks in the trajectory model need to be modified for service to such other severely disabled groups as the mentally ill or frail elderly?

IMPLICATIONS FOR OTHER AREAS
OF ENVIRONMENTAL PRACTICE

The six areas of environmental practice that were the focus of this book are somewhat limited in terms of the potential domain for this kind of practice. Some of the other areas that could be included are specific intervention areas such as the practice of normalization, the community, and interventions in various substantive social problem arenas such as unemployment, adult and child welfare, housing, the mentally ill, the developmentally disabled, and the frail elderly. Although these social problem areas have been used here to illustrate general environmental practice interventions, they have particular characteristics that require more specialized knowledge and skill. For example, the principles and skills associated with normalization were initially developed for the field of mental retardation, but they are now being applied to service for the mentally ill. These principles are probably also relevant for other vulnerable populations; however, although normalization concepts may be generalizable to several areas of environmental practice, their application to specific substantive social problems requires specialized knowledge of tht particular area.

Also, the community as an arena for environmental practice has much potential. "Community work" gained prominence in Great Britain (Thomas 1983). In this book, the community has been mentioned as an important element and particularly relevant for resource coordination and social support. The community is seen as the *cause* and *solution* of social problems. "It is only by creating a community that we establish a basis for commitment, obligation, and social support" (Specht and Courtney 1994:27). The community as a *target* for intervention to strengthen its capacities to solve problems has traditionally been the province of community organization and planning. The poverty programs in the 1960s used the community as the foundation for practice (Neugeboren 1970b). Community-based service-delivery models are receiving renewed interest as a strategy for ameliorating social problems (Rothman 1994; Specht and Courtney 1994:152-175). This is another fruitful area for environmental practice.

These areas for potential application of the knowledge and skills of environmental practice are interconnected. For example, the housing resource area affects on child abuse, the mentally ill, the developmentally disabled, and the frail elderly. Therefore, environmental practice in the housing area would be critical for the human services. Employment is another fruitful area for environmental practice, since it also impacts on other social problem areas, such as welfare and rehabilitation of the mentally ill.

INTEGRATION OF MICRO AND MACRO PRACTICE

Implications for Service Delivery

The integration of micro and macro practice was presented as a basic ingredient of environmental practice. The common knowledge and skills shared by these levels of intervention, as well as their interdependencies, have implications for the design of human-service delivery programs. Role definitions and relations between direct-service workers, community organizers, and administrators, planners, and policymakers will need to be redefined to enable better communication and allow closer collaboration.

Implications for Education and Training

The integration of micro and macro practice has implications for in-service training, which traditionally separates instruction for these levels. The same is true for specialized professional education programs. In both training and formal education, classes will have to be integrated to include persons from both levels of practice, as is currently done in generalist education. However, we must be cautious not to negate the *differences* between these two practice levels. The goal of education and training is to facilitate closer collaboration because both practice levels need each other in order to accomplish their shared objectives.

Implications for Research

Study of the collaboration of micro and macro practice would enhance understanding of the opportunities and constraints in this type of endeavor. The consequences for service users of this kind of cooperative effort is another potential area for research.

CONCLUSIONS

A three-dimensional model for environmental practice is proposed that integrates the micro and macro levels in the organizational, community, and societal arenas with six common practice skills. The social context of practice is recognized as an important element in service intervention. Thus, the environment is presented as the *context* as well as the *target* of practice. Understanding the distinction between practice contexts and targets is viewed as basic to successful environmental practice.

In conclusion, environmental practice is advocated as an important area that needs further development to allow the human services to respond to the needs of vulnerable populations. This is in line with Specht and Courtney's (1994) prescription of the mission for social work in the twenty-first century: "Building a community based system of social care" by helping individuals make use of their social resources (23).

Recognition that environmental practice is a "central and essential tradition in social work" was acknowledged by the editor of *Social Work* (Hartman 1990:373). To accomplish this we would need to "overcome the social work rhetoric that claims to address environmental problems while dealing with psychological matters" (Morris 1989:478-479). We can learn from the community social work model developed in England (Harrison 1989:73-75). A call has gone out for social workers to organize professionally for this type of socially oriented practice, as was done by psychologists and sociologists after World War II (Neugeboren 1990:373-374). The favorable climate environmentalism provides the human services with the opportunity to recapture their historic mission of better serving service consumer needs by facilitating more-benevolent service milieus.

Appendix

AGENCY PROFILE OUTLINE

I. *Type of Agency* (federal, state, community, or neighborhood-service agency).

II. *Operational Description of Agency.*

1. Service mandate.

2. Funding source.

3. Structure (including actual personnel).

   • Hierarchy of authority (who makes decisions?).

   • Hiring procedures–Case or workload distribution.

4. Service pattern (intake care and end service).

   Description of how clients get into system, procedures followed in delivering services, how cases are terminated.

   • Accountability system.

   • Recording of unmet needs.

   • Specification of eligibility requirements, length of service and its nature.

   • If there is multidisciplinary approach, on who is ultimately responsible for what decisions are made in behalf of client?

5. Ideology.

   • Particular client problems and population.

6. Identification of service gaps and any services that would be complementary.

- Lack of service.

- Estimated services (waiting lists).

- Service "negotiation" problems (what kind of service we may provide to an agency and how their services are needed for our clientele).

AFFILIATION AGREEMENT FOR AGENCIES PARTICIPATING IN THE COUNTY UNIFIED SERVICE SYSTEM

The purpose of this agreement is to formalize the_____

(name of agency)

commitment to become a member of the County Unified Service System (CUSS).

By this agreement, I,_____ , as a duly authorized representative of_____ agree that maximum

(name of agency)

utilization of community resources is a prerequisite for the attainment of our goals to improve individual and family functioning in the community. The establishment of a comprehensive community social service system is seen as a necessity for the provision of relevant and effective services to our mutual clients. Toward this end, we agree to facilitate the coordination of our services at the case level, and to engage in an exchange of resources whenever there is an opportunity to develop joint programs, provided that such programs will enhance the attainment of each agency's goals. We recognize that a client's interests are best served when clear lines of communication and responsibility between service providers are delineated.

We further agree that the use and expansion of natural and community supports e.g., family and friends) for individuals and families have more long-lasting benefits than the time-limited relief provided by governmental and private providers. For these reasons, we agree to help each other in the active search for community-based, leas- restrictive solutions to individual and family problems.

In consideration of our affiliation, each agency agrees as follows:

I. To develop and sign an affiliation agreement with each other for the purpose of organizing our service delivery around the service needs of the community. This agreements will define mutually agreed upon roles and responsibilities of each agency to provide individuals and families known to both affiliated agencies with a coordinated intervention approach.

II. To develop, sign, and implement liaison procedures for inter-agency collaboration. Liaison procedural agreements will serve to maximize the use of available resources and to resolve interdisciplinary conflicts that may arise between agency officials during the process of ad-hoc referrals and staffing of cases. The designated liaison will contribute to the development of a centralized Resource Data Bank system. The liaison agreements should be preceded by a detailed description of the participating agency's structure and service-delivery process. These "Agency Service Profiles" will serve as the basis for the development of specific procedures for interagency intervention. These procedures, which include the agency service profile, will be filed in the Resource Data Bank, where they will be available to all the staff of the affiliated agencies.

III. To seek out opportunities to develop joint programs that provide for interdisciplinary forums. These programs will be designed to maximize agencies' effectiveness in working together toward the solution of clients' social problems. One way to enhance interagency effectiveness is through cross training, whereby individuals or groups from each agency visit another affiliated agency to share service availability and the eligibility requirements of their agencies. As a member of the CUSS, we agree to participate in the development and improvement of a joint monthly calendar of cross training activities.

IV. To meet once a month or as frequently as decided by the members to:

1. Report on our individual agency's activities and progress toward the establishment of a comprehensive CUSS.

2. Plan activities and programs designed to enhance interagency coordination.

The scope of this agreement is limited to the procedural relationships between the parties to this agreement for the provision of services to mutual clients, or potential clients and is subject to all laws concerning client's rights and confidentiality, and the policies and procedures of the agencies involved. This agreement is subject to renegotiation at any time there is a policy change that impacts on the agencies' abilities to fulfill the terms of the agreement.

_____ _____ _____

AGENCY   EXECUTIVE DIRECTOR   DATE

Bibliography

Abel, E. M. and K. J. Kazmerski. 1994. Protecting the inclusion of macro content in generalist practice. *Journal of Community Practice* 1(3):59-72.

Abrams, P. 1980. Social change, social networks and neighborhood care. *Social Work Services* 22:12-23.

Ad'Hoc Committee on Advocacy. 1969. The social worker as advocate: Champion of social victims. *Social Work* 14(2):16-22.

Aiken, M., R. Dewar, N. DiTomaso, J. Hage, and G. Zeitz. 1975. *Coordinating human services: New strategies for building service delivery systems.* San Francisco: Jossey-Bass.

Anderson, G. A., Jr. 1985. The assessment of systems in promoting collaborative aftercare: Religious and mental health organizations in partnership. *The Journal of Pastoral Care* 39(3):236-248.

Anderson, S. V. and E. Bauwens. 1981. *Chronic health problems.* St. Louis: Mosby.

Anthony, W. A. 1979. The rehabilitation approach to diagnosis. In *Community support for the long-term patient.* New Directions for Mental Health Services No. 2. San Francisco: Jossey-Bass.

Anthony, W. A., M. R. Cohen, and B. F. Cohen. 1984. Psychiatric rehabilitation. In *The chronic mental patient,* ed. J. A. Talbott. New York: Grune & Stratton.

Anthony, W. A. and R. P. Lieberman. 1986. The practice of psychiatric rehabilitation: Historical, conceptual, and research base. *Schizophrenia Bulletin* 12(4):542-559.

Anthony, W. A. and M. Jansen. 1984. Predicting the vocational capacity of the chronically mentally ill. *American Psychologist* 39(5) 537-544.

Anthony, W. A., P. Nemec, and M. Cohen. 1987. Assessment in psychiatric rehabilitation. *Handbook of measurement and evaluation in rehabilitation,* ed. B. Bolten. Baltimore: Paul Brookes.

Argyris, C. R., R. Putnam, and D. M. Smith. 1985. *Action science.* San Francisco: Jossey-Bass.

Atkins, R. C. 1988. *Dr. Atkins' health revolution: How complementary medicine can extend your life*. New York: Houghton Mifflin.

Auslander, W. F., J. Bubb, M. Rogge, and J. V. Sontage. 1993. Family stress and resources: Potential areas of intervention in children recently diagnosed with diabetes. *Health and Social Work* 18(2):101-113.

Auslander, G. K. and H. Litwin. 1987. The parameters of network intervention: A social work application. *Social Service Review* 61(2):303-318.

Austin, C. D. 1981. Client assessment in context. *Social Work Research and Abstracts* 17:4-12.

Austin, C. D. 1983. Case management in long-term care: Options and opportunities. *Health and Social Work* 8(1):16-30.

Austin, D., P. Caragone, J. Nix, M. Campos, A. Hardesty, J. Neely, and P. Potter. 1980. An analysis of the function of the case manager in five mental health social service settings. Case Management Research Project. Austin, TX: School of Social Work, University of Texas, Austin.

Austin, M. J. 1981. *Supervisory management in the human services.* Englewood Cliffs, NJ: Prentice-Hall.

Austin, M. J. 1986. Community organization and social administration: Partnership or irrelevance? *Administration in Social Work* 10(3):27-39.

Austin, M. J. and R. Patti. 1984. *Environmental intervention in human service practice*. Seattle, WA: University of Washington School of Social Work. Mimeograph.

Aviram, U. 1990. Community care of the seriously mentally ill: Continuing problems and current issues. *Community Mental Health Journal* 26(1):69-87.

Aviram, U. and J. Katan. 1991. Preferences of social workers: Prestige scales of populations, services and methods in social work. *International Social Work Journal* 34(1): 37-55.

Aviram, U. and S. Segal. 1973. Exclusion of the mentally ill: A reflection of an old problem. *Archives of General Psychiatry* 23(2):120-131.

Azzarto, J. 1992. Medicalization of the problems of the elderly. In *Case management and social work practice*, ed. S. M. Rose. New York: Longman.

Balgopal, P. R. 1989. Occupational social work: An expanded client perspective. *Social Work* 34(5):437-442.

Ballew, J. R. 1985. Role of natural helpers in preventing child abuse and neglect. *Social Work*, 30(1):37-41.

Ballew, J. R. and G. Mink. 1986. *Case management in the human services*. Springfield, IL: Charles Thomas.

Barker, R. et al. 1978. *Habitats, environments and human behavior.* San Francisco: Jossey-Bass.

Baumheier, E. C. 1982. Services integration in the field of health and human services. In *Health services integration: Lessons for the 1980's*. Volume 4. Washington, DC: Institute of Medicine, National Academy of Sciences.

Baxter, R., R. Applebaum, J. Callahan, Jr., J. B. Christianson, and S. L. Day. 1983. *The planning and implementation of channelling: Early experiences of the national long-term care demonstration.* Princeton: Mathematica.

Bayley, M. J. 1973. *Mental health handicap and community care.* London: Routledge, Kegan, Paul.

Beatrice, D. F. 1981. Case management: A policy for long-term care. In *Reforming the long-term care system: Financial and organizational options,* ed. J. J. Callahan and S. S. Wallack. Lexington, MA: D.C. Heath.

Beattie, M. 1987. *Codependent no more*. New York: Harper & Row.

Beels, C. C., L. Gutworth, J. Berkley, and E. Struening. 1984. Measurement of social support. *Schizophrenia Bull.* 10(399-411).

Berger, C. S. and K. B. Nash. 1984. Developing roles for the macro practitioner within the health field. *Administration in Social Work* 8:67-76.

Berkowitz, R., L. Kuipers, Eberlein-Frief, and J. Leff. 1981. Lowering expressed emotions in relatives of schizophrenics. In *New developments in interventions with families of schizophrenics,* ed. M. J. Goldstein. San Francisco: Jossey-Bass.

Biegel, D., R. Schultz, B. Shore, and E. Gordon. 1989. Economic supports for family caregivers of the elderly: Public sector policies. *Family involvement in the treatment of the frail elderly,* ed. M. Z. Goldstein. Washington, DC: American Psychiatric Press.

Biegel, D. E., A. K. Shore, and E. Gordon. 1984. *Building support networks for the elderly.* Beverly Hills, CA: Sage.

Biegel, D. E. and A. Blum. 1990. *Aging and caregiving.* Newbury Park, CA: Sage.

Biegel, D. E., E. Sales, and R. Schultz. 1991. *Family caregiving in chronic illness.* Newbury Park, CA: Sage.

Black, R. B., D. H. Dornan, and J. P. Allegrante. 1986. Challenges in developing health promotion services for the chronically mentally ill. *Social Work* 31(4):287-293.

Blair, S. N., P. V. Piserchia, C. S. Wilbur, and J. H. Crowder. 1986. A public health intervention model for work-site health promotion. *Journal of American Medical Association* 155(7):921-926.

Bly, J. L., R. C. Jones, and J. E. Richardson. 1986. Impact of worksite health promotion on health care costs and utilization. *Journal of American Medical Association* 256(23):3235-3240.

Bosk, C. 1979. *Forgive and remember: Managing medical failure.* Chicago: University of Chicago Press.

Brager, G. and S. Holloway. 1978. *Changing human service organizations: Politics and practice.* New York: Free Press.

Brawley, E. A. 1985. The mass media: A vital adjunct to the new community and administrative practice. *Administration in Social Work* 9(4):63-74.

Briar, S. and B. J. Blythe. 1985. Agency support for evaluating the outcome of social work services. *Administration in Social Work* 9(2):25-36.

Brieland, D. 1990. The hull house tradition and the contemporary social worker: Was Jane Adams really a social worker? *Social Work* 35(2): 134-140.

Brody, E. 1981. Women in the middle and family help to older people. *The Gerontologist* 21:471-480.

Brower, A. M. 1988. Can the ecological model guide social work practice? *Social Service Review* 62(3):411-429.

Brown, G. E. 1966. The public relations function of the administrator. In *Public relations in health and welfare,* ed. Frances Schmidt and Harold Weiner. New York: Columbia University Press.

Brown, G. W., J. L. Birley, and J. K. Wing. 1972. Influence of family life on the course of schizophrenic disorders: A replication. *British Journal of Psychiatry* 121:241-258.

Butler, A. C. 1990. A re-evaluation of social work students career interests. *Journal of Social Work Education* 26(1):45-56.

Callan, D., J. Garrison, and E. Zerger. 1975. Working with the families and social networks of drug abusers. *Journal of Psychedelic Drugs* 7:19-25.

Camasso, M. J. and A. E. Camasso. 1986. Social supports, undesirable life events and psychological distress in a disadvantaged population. *Social Service Review* 60(3):378-394.

Campbell, A. 1981. *The sense of well-being in America.* New York: McGraw-Hill.

Caplan, G. 1964. *Principles of preventive psychiatry.* New York: Basic Books.

Carter, R. K. 1987. Measuring client outcomes: The experience of the states. *Administration in Social Work* 11(3/4):73-88.

Chambers, D. L. 1975. Community based treatment and the constitution: The principle of least restrictive alternative. In *Alternatives to mental hospital treatment,* ed. L. J. Stein and M. A. Test. New York: Plenum Press.

Cheung, K. M. 1988. Home care services for the elderly: Cost savings implications to Medicaid. *Social Service Review* 62(1):127-136.

Clark, D. W. and T. F. Williams (eds.). 1976. *Teaching of chronic illness and aging.* Washington, DC: DHEW Publication No. (NIH) 75-876.

Clark, H. 1988. State of the neighborhood. Report of citizens committee for the city of New York.

Cloward, R. A. 1959. Illegitimate means, anomie and deviant behavior. *American Sociological Review* 24: 166-176.

Cnaan, R. A., L. Blankertz, K. Messinger, and J. R. Gardner. 1989. Psychosocial rehabilitation: Towards a theoretical base. *Psychosocial Rehabilitation Journal* 11(1):33-56.

Cnaan, R. A., L. Blankertz, K. Messinger, and J. R. Gardner. 1988. Psychosocial Rehabilitation: Toward a definition. *Psychosocial Rehabilitation Journal,* 13(1):33-56.

Cocozzelli, C. and C. G. Hudson. 1989. Recent advances in alcohol diagnosis and treatment assessment research: Implications for practice. *Social Service Review* 63(4):533-552

Cohen, F. and R. S. Lazarus. 1979. Coping with the stress of illness. In *Health psychology–A handbook,* ed. G. C. Stone, F. Cohen, and N. E. Adler. San Francisco: Jossey-Bass.

Cohen, M. R., R. L. Vitalo, W. A. Anthony, R. M. Pierce, 1980. *The skills of community service coordination.* Psychiatric rehabilitation practice series: Book 6. Baltimore: University Park Press.

Collins, A. H. and D. Pancoast. 1976. *Naturally helping networks.* Washington, DC: National Association of Social Workers.

Commission on Chronic Illness. 1956. *Care of the long-term patient.* Cambridge, MA: Harvard University Press.

Corbin, J. M. and A. Strauss. 1988. *Unending work and care.* San Francisco. CA: Jossey-Bass.

Council on Social Work Education (CSWE). 1992. *Curriculum Policy Statement for Masters & Baccalaureate Degree Programs in Social Work.* Washington, DC. CSWE.

Cowen, E. L. 1982. Help is where you find it: Four informal helping groups. *American Psychologist* 37:385-395.

Cox, C. 1992. Expanding social work's role in home care: An ecological perspective. *Social Work* 37(2):179-183.

Cox, E. O., R. J. Parsons, and P. J. Kimboko. 1988. Social services and international caregivers: Issues for social work. *Social Work* 33(5):430-434.

Crotty, P. and R. Kulys. 1985. Social support networks: The view of schizophrenic clients and their significant others. *Social Work* 30(5):301-309.

Cummings, E. 1968. *Systems of social regulation.* New York: Atherton.

Curtin, M. and I. Lubkin. 1986. What is chronicity? In *Chronic illness: Impact and intervention,* ed. I. Lubkin. Boston: Jones and Bartlett.

D'Augelli, A. R., T. R. Vallance, S. J. Danish, C. E. Young, and J. L. Gerdes. 1981. The community helpers project: A description of a prevention strategy for rural communities. *Journal of Prevention* 1:209-224.

David, T., R. Moos, and J. Kahn. 1981. Community integration among elderly residents of sheltered care settings. *American Journal of Community Psychology* 9:513-526.

Devore, W. and E. G. Schlesinger. 1981. *Ethnic sensitive social work practice*. St. Louis: Mosby.

De Weaver, K. L. 1983. Deinstitutionalization of the developmentally disabled: A challenge to social work. 28(6):435-439.

Di Matteo, M. R. and R. Hays. 1981. Social support and serious illness. In Social networks and social support, ed. B. H. Gottlieb. Beverly Hill, CA: Sage.

Dickerson, M. U. 1981. *Social work practice with the mentally retarded*. New York: Free Press.

Doane, J. A. 1977. A mental health training and consultation program for family practice attorneys. Unpublished manuscript, Los Angeles: University of California-Los Angeles.

Douglas, A. 1962. *Industrial peacemaking*. New York: Columbia University Press.

Dunphy, J. 1984. For the elderly, No place like home. *Detroit Free Press*, May, 15, 1b, 3b.

East, E. 1992. Family as resource: Maintaining chronically mentally ill members in the community. *Health and Social Work* 17(2):93-98.

Ehlers, W. H., M. J. Austin, J. C. Prothero. 1976. *Administration for the human services*. New York: Harper & Row.

Ephross, P. and M. Reisch. 1982. The ideology of some social work texts. *Social Service Review* 56(1):273-281.

Epstein, I. 1981. Advocates on advocacy: An exploratory study. *Social Work Research and Abstracts* 17(2):5-12.

Ewalt, P. L. and R. M. Honeyfield. 1981. Needs of persons in long term care. *Social Work* 26(3):221-223.

Ezell, M. and R. J. Patti. 1990. State human service agencies: Structure and organization. *Social Service Review* 64(1):22-45.

Fairweather, G. 1969. *Community life for the mentally ill*. Hawthorne, NY: Aldine.

Falloon, I. R., J. L. Boyd, and C. W. McGill. 1984. *Family care of schizophrenia*. New York: Guilford Press.

Families Anonymous. 1977. A basic pamphlet. Post Office Box 528, Van Nuys, California, 91408.

Family Development Act. 1992. Chapter 523. Laws of New Jersey, 1991.

Family Support Act. 1988. P. L. 100-485. U.S.C. 1305.

Family Support Act. 1993. Bill No. A2938. New Jersey State Legislature.

Family Support and Preservation Act. 1993. L. 1993, chapter 157.

Feldman, L. 1991. Evaluating the impact of intensive family preservation services in New Jersey. In *Family preservation services: Research and evaluation,* ed. K. Wells and D. Biegel, Newbury Park, CA: Sage.

Fellin, P. 1987. *The community and the social worker.* Itaska, IL: Peacock.

Ferris, P. A. and C. A. Marshall. 1987. A model project for families of the chronically mentally ill. *Social Work* 32(2):110-114.

Fiorentine, R. and O. Grusky. 1990. When case managers manage the seriously mentally ill; A role contingency approach. *Social Service Review* 64(1):79-93.

Fischer, J. 1973. Is casework effective? A review. *Social Work* 18(1):5-20.

Fischer, J. 1978. *Effectiveness practice: An eclectic approach.* New York: McGraw-Hill.

Fleishman, E. A. and D. R. Peters. 1962. Interpersonal values, leadership attitudes and managerial success. *Personnel Psychology* 15:126-143.

Frankel, H. 1988. Family-centered, home based services in child protection: A review of the research. *Social Service Review* 62(1):137-157.

Fredericks, C. 1981. *Arthritis: Don't learn to live with it.* New York: Putnam.

Freeman, H. and O. Simmons. 1963. *The mental patient comes home.* New York John Wiley & Sons Inc.

Fried. M. 1963. Grieving for a lost home. In *The urban condition,* ed. L. J. Duhl. New York: Basic Books.

Froland, C., D. Pancoast, N. Chapman, and P. J. Kimboko. 1981. *Helping networks and human services.* Beverly Hills, CA: Sage

Galaskiewicz, J. 1979. *Exchange networks and community politics.* Beverly Hills, CA: Sage.

Gans, H. J. 1963. Social and physical planning for the elimination of urban poverty. *Washington University Law Quarterly* 1:2-18.

Garbarino, J. 1977. The human ecology of child maltreatment: A conceptual model for research. *Journal of Marriage and the Faily*, 39:721-726.

Garbarino, J. P. 1980. Preventing maltreatment. In *Prevention in mental health*. Vol 1. ed. R. Price. Beverly Hills: Sage.

Garbarino, J. S., S. H. Stocking, and Associates. 1980. *Protecting children from abuse and neglect*. San Francisco: Jossey-Bass.

Garrison, J. 1974. Network techniques: Case studies in the screening-linking-planning conference method. *Family Process* 13:337-354.

Garvin, C. and N. A. Seabury, 1984. *Interpersonal practice in social work*. Englewood Cliffs, NJ: Prentice-Hall.

Geiss, G. R. and N. Viswanathn (eds.). 1986. *The human edge: Information technology and helping people*. New York: The Haworth Press.

Genkins, M. 1985. Strategic planning for social work marketing. *Administration in Social Work* 9(10):35-46.

Germain, C. B. 1973. An ecological perspective in social work. *Social Casework* 54(6):323-330.

Germain, C. B. 1994. Using an ecological perpective. In *Practice with highly vulnerable clients*, ed. J. Rothman. Englewood Cliffs, NJ: Prentice-Hall.

Germain, C. B. and A. Gitterman. 1980. *The life model of social work practice*. New York: Columbia University Press.

Gibelman, M. 1983. Social work education and the changing nature of public agency practice. *Journal of Education for Social Work* 19:21-28.

Gilbert, N. 1982. Policy issues in primary prevention. *Social Work* 27(4): 293-297.

Gilbert, N., H. Miller, and H. Specht. 1980. *An introduction to social work practice*. Englewood Cliffs: Prentice-Hall.

Gilbert, N. and H. Specht. 1974. *Dimensions of social welfare policy*. Englewood Cliffs, NJ: Prentice-Hall.

Glasser, P. H. and C. D. Garvin. 1977. Social group work: The organizational and environmental approach. *Encyclopedia of Social Work*, 1338-1350. Washington, DC: N.A.S.W.

Glastonbury, B. 1985. *Computers in social work*. London: Macmillan.

Goffman, E. 1961. *Asylums*. Garden City, NY: Doubleday.

Goffman, E. 1963. *Stigma: Notes on the management of spoiled identity.* Englewood Cliffs, NJ: Prentice-Hall.

Goldberg, E. M. and T. Warburton. 1979. *End and means in social work.* London: Allen and Unwin.

Goleman, D. 1986. Focus on day-to-day support offers hope to schizophrenics. *The New York Times,* March 19, B-12.

Gottlieb, B. H. 1983. *Social support strategies: Guidelines for mental health practice.* Beverly Hills, CA: Sage.

Gottlieb, B. H. 1985. Assessing and strengthening the impact of social support on mental health. *Social Work* 30:293-300.

Goudenough, W. H. 1963. *Cooperation in change.* New York: Russell Sage Foundation.

Grant. G. and C. Wenger. 1983. Patterns of partnership: Three modes of care for the elderly. In *Rediscovery of Self Help*, ed. D. L. Pancoast, P. Parker, and C. Froland. Beverly Hills, CA: Sage

Grasso, A. J. and I. Epstein. 1987. Management by measurement: Organizational dilemmas and opportunities. *Administration in Social Work* 11(3/4):89-100.

Grinnell, R. M., Jr. 1973. Environmental modification: Casework's concern or casework's neglect. *Social Service Review* 47:208-220.

Grinnell, R. M., Jr. and N. S. Kyte. 1974. Modifying the environment. *Social Work* 19(4):477-483.

Grinnell, R. M., Jr. and N. Kyte. 1975. Environmental modification: A study. *Social Work* 20(4):313-318.

Guillemin, J., and L. Holstrom. 1986. *Mixed blessings: Intensive care for newborns.* New York: Oxford University Press.

Gummer, B. 1990. *The politics of social administration: Managing organizational politics in social agencies.* Englewood Cliffs: Prentice-Hall.

Gutheil, I. A. 1992. Considering the physical environment: An essential component of good practice. *Social Work* 37(5):391-397.

Hackett, T. P. 1978. The use of groups in the rehabilitation of the postcoronary patient. *Advances in Cardiology* 24:127-135.

Hagen, J. L. 1992. Woman, work, and welfare: Is there a role for social work? *Social Work* 37(1):9-1.

Hagen, J. L. 1994. JOBS and case management in 10 states. *Social Work* 39(2):197-206.

Hagen, J. L. and L. Wang. 1993. roes and functions of public welfare workers. *Administration in Social Work* 17(2):81-103.

Hall, R. 1977. *Organizations: Structuure and process.* 3d. ed. Englewood Cliffs, NJ: Prentice-Hall.

Harkness, L. and P. Mulinski. 1988. Performance standards for social workers. *Social Work* 33(4):339-344.

Harrison, R. K. 1979. The doctor patient relationship: The physician as a mental health resource. Unpublished doctoral dissertation, Dept. of Psychology, State University of New York, Buffalo.

Harrison, W. D. 1987. Reflective practice in social care. *Social Service Review* 61(3):393-404.

Harrison, W. D. 1989. Social work and the search for post-industrial community. *Social Work* 34(1):73-75.

Harrison, W. D. and G. Hoshino. 1985. Britain's Barclay report: Lessons for the United States. *Social Work* 29:215.

Hartman, A. 1990. Editor's note. *Environmental Practice Social Work* 35(4):373.

Hartman, A. 1989. Homelessness: Public issue and private trouble. *Social Work* 34(6):483-484.

Hasenfeld, Y. 1972. People processing organizations: An exchange approach. *American Sociological Review* 37:135, 256-263.

Hasenfeld, Y. 1983. *Human service organizations.* Englewood Cliffs, NJ: Prentice-Hall.

Hermone, R. H. 1974. How to negotiate and come out the winner. *Management Review* 1:19-25.

Hersey, P. and K. Blanchard. 1977. *Management of organizational behavior: Utilizing human resources.* 3d. ed. Englewood Cliffs, NJ: Prentice-Hall.

Hoch, C. and G. C. Hemmens. 1987. Linking informal and formal help: Conflict along a continuum of care. *Social Service Review* 61(3):432-446.

Holcomb, B. 1988. The druggist's new role: Today's pharmacist must help people monitor their use of medication. *New York Times Magazine,* April 17, Section 6, Part 2, 39.

Holcomb, W. 1985. *Building a support system: Manuao for the development of church, synagogue and mental health agency.* Sponsored support programs for long-term recipients of mental health services. New Jersey Division of Mental Health and Hospitals.

Holloway, S. and G. Brager. 1985. Implicit negotiating and organizational practice. *Administration in Social Work* 9(2):15-24.

Hopps, G. H. 1986. The catch in social support. *Social Work* 31(6):419-420.

Hudson, C. G. 1990. The performance of state community mental health systems: A path model. *Social Service Review* 64(1):94-120.

Hudson, W. W. 1987. Measuring clinical outcomes and their use for managers. *Administration in Social Work* 11(3/4):59-72.

Illich, I. 1976. *Medical nemesis.* New York: Random House.

Indik, B. and F. Berrien. 1968. *People, groups and organizations.* New York: Teachers College Press.

Inglehart, A. P. 1990. Discharge planning: Professional perspectives versus organizational effects. *Health and Social Work* 15(4):301-309.

Iodice, J. D. and J. S. Wodarski. 1987. Aftercare treatment for schizophrenics living at home. *Social Work* 32(2):122-128.

Jansson, B. 1984. *Theory and practice of social welfare policy: Analysis, processes and current issues.* Belmont, CA: Wadsworth.

Jarrett, R. B. and J. A. Fairbanks. 1987. Psychologist's views: APA's advocacy and resource expenditures on social and profesional issues. *Professional Psychology: Research and Practice* 18(6): 643-646.

Johnson, L. C. 1995. *Social work practice: A generalist approach.* 5th Edition. Boston, MA: Allyn and Bacon.

Johnson, P. and R. Rubin. 1983. Case management in mental health: A social work domain. *Social Work* 28(1):49-55.

Judge, K. and J. Smith. 1983. *Who volunteers.* Personal Social Services Research Unit, discussion paper 267. University of Kent at Canterbury.

Kadushin, A. 1976. *Supervision in social work.* New York: Columbia University Press.

Kahn, A. J. 1969. *Theory and practice of social planning.* New York: Russell Sage.

Kam-Fong Monit Cheung. 1988. Home care services for the elderly: Cost saving implications for medicine. *Social Service Review* 62(1):127-136.

Kane, R. 1980. Discharge planning: An undischarged responsibility. *Health and Social Work* 5:2-3.

Kane, R. A. 1992. Case management: Ethical pitfalls on the road to high quality managed care. In *Case management and social work practice*, ed. S. P. Rose. New York: Longman.

Kane, R. A. and R. L. Kane. 1984. *Assessing the elderly*. Lexington, MA: Lexington Books.

Kanter, J. 1985. Case management of the young adult chronic patient: A clinical perspective. In *Clinical issues in treating the chronically mentally ill*, ed. J. S. Kanter. San Francisco: Jossey-Bass.

Kanter, J. 1987. Mental health case management: A professional domain. *Social Work* 32(5):461-462.

Karls, J. M. and K. Wandrei. 1994. *PIE: Person-in-environment system*. Washington, DC: NASW Press.

Karrass, C. L. 1970. *The negotiating game*. New York: Crowell.

Katz, D. and R. Kahn. 1978. *Social psychology of organizations*. New York: John Wiley & Sons, Inc.

Kaye, L. W. 1985. Home care for the aged: A fragile partnership. *Social Work* 30:312-317.

Kaye, L. W. 1994. The effectiveness of services marketing: Perception of executive directors of gerontological programs. *Administration in Social Work* 18(2):69-86.

Kennedy, M. 1980. *Office politics*. New York: Warner Books.

Kettner, P. M. and L. L. Martin. 1985. Issues in the development of marketing systems for purchase of service contracting. *Administration in Social Work* 9(3):69-82.

Kirk, S. A. and Greenley, J. R. 1974. Denying or delivering services? *Social Work* 19:439-447.

Kirst-Ashman, K. K. and G. H. Hull, Jr. 1993. *Understanding generalist practice*. Chicago, IL.: Nelson Hall.

Knight, R. C. 1980. Environmental evaluation research: Evaluator roles and inherent social commitments. *Environment and Behavior* 12:520-532.

Kolata, G. 1994. Wrong drugs given to 1 in 4 elderly. *The New York Times*, July 27, C8.

Kroeber, D. and H. Watson. 1979. Is there a best MIS department location? *Information Management* 12:165-173.

Kruzich, J. M. 1988. The chronically mentally ill in nursing homes: Policy and practice issues. *Health and Social Work* 13(5):553-564.

Kruzich, J. M. and W. Berg. 1985. Predictors of self sufficiency for the mentally ill in long term care. *Community Mental Health Journal* 21(3):198-207.

Kruzich, J. M. and B. J. Friesen. 1984. Blending administrative and community organization practice: The case of community residential facilities. *Administration in Social Work* 8:55-66.

Kurtz, L. F. 1984. Linking treatment centers with alcoholics anonymous. *Social Work in Health Care* 9:85-94.

Kutz, L., K. B. Mann, and A. Chambon. 1987. Linking between social workers and mental health mutual-aid groups. *Social Work in Health Care* 13(1):69-76.

Lamb, H. R. 1980. Therapist-case managers: More than brokers of services. *Hospital and Community Psychiatry* 31(11):762-764.

Lamb, H. R. and V. Goertzel. 1972. High expectations of long term ex-state hospital patients. *American Journal of Psychiatry* 129: 421-475.

Lamb, H. R. and R. Peele. 1984. The need for continuing asylum and sanctuary. *Hospital and Community Psychiatry* 38(8):798-802.

Lanoil, J. 1980. The chronically mentally ill in the community-case management models. *Psychosocial Rehabilitation Journal* 4(2):1-6.

Larkin, J. P. and B. M. Hopcroft. 1993. In-hospital respite as a moderator of caregiver stress. *Health and Social Work* 18(2):132-138.

Lauffer, A. 1978. *Social planning on the community level.* Englewood Cliffs, NJ: Prentice-Hall.

Lauffer, A. 1982. *Getting the resources you need.* Sage Human Services Guides, Volume 26. Beverly Hills, CA: Sage.

Lauffer, A. 1984. *Strategic marketing for non-for profit organizations.* New York: Free Press.

Lauffer, A. 1986. To market to market: A nuts and bolts approach to strategic planning in human service organizations. *Administration in Social Work* 10(4):31-40.

Lauffer, A., L. Nybell, C. Overberger, B. Reed, and L. Zeff. 1977.

Understanding your social agency. Vol. 3. Human Service Guides. Beverly Hills: Sage.

Lechner, V. M. 1993. Support systems and stress reduction among workers caring for dependent parents. *Social Work* 3(4):461-469.

Levine, I. S. and M. Fleming. 1985. *Human resource development: Issues in case management.* Rockville, MD: Office of State and Community Liaison, National Institute of Mental Health.

Levy, L. 1982. Issues in research and evaluation. In *The self help revolution*, ed. A. Gartner and F. Reesman. New York: Human Sciences.

Lewis, J. and M. Lewis. 1983. *Management of human service programs.* Monterey, CA: Brooks-Cole.

Lindemann, E. 1944. Symptomatology and management of acute grief. *American Journal of Psychiatry* 101:141-148.

Linsk, N. L., S. E. Osterbusch, L. Simon-Rusinowitz, and S. M. Keigher. 1988. Community agency support of family caregiving. *Health and Social Work* 13(3):209-218.

Lister, L. 1987. Contemporary direct practice roles. *Social Work* 32(5):384-391.

Litwak, E. and H. J. Meyer,. 1966. A balance theory of coordination between bureaucratic organizations and community primary groups. *Administrative Science Quarterly* 11:21-58.

Litwak, E. and J. Rothman. 1970. Toward the theory and practice of coordination between formal organizations. In *Organizations and clients: Essays on the sociology of service*, ed. W. Rosengren and M. Lefton. Columbus, OH: Bobbs Merrill.

Litwin, H. 1985. Community care capacity: A view from Israel. In *Support networks in a caring community*, ed. J. A Yoder, J. M. L. Jonker, and R. A. B. Leaper. Dordrecht/Boston/Lancaster: Martius Nijhoff.

Logigian, E. L., R. F. Kaplan, and A. C. Steere. 1990. Chronic neurological manifestations of lyme disease. *The New England Journal of Medicine* 323(21):1438-1443.

Lowenberg, F. 1981. The destigmitization of public dependency. *Social Service Review* 5(2):434-452.

Lowy, L. 1985. *The implications of demographic trends as they affect the elderly.* Paper presented at the 25th Annual Scientific

Meeting of the Boston Society of Gerontologic Psychiatry, Boston, MA.

Lubkin, I. M. 1986. *Chronic illness: Impact and interventions*. Boston: Jones and Bartlett.

Lucas, H. C., Jr. 1975. *Why Information Systems Fail*. New York: Columbia University Press.

Maguire, L. 1983. *Understanding social networks.* Sage Human Service Guide 32. Beverly Hills, CA: Sage.

Maluccio, A. N. 1981. *Promoting competence in clients*. New York: Free Press.

Manoleas, P. 1992. Should social workers accept a disease model of substance abuse? Yes. In *Controversial issues in social work*, ed. E. Gambrill and R. Pruger. Needham Heights, MA: Allyyn and Bacon.

March, J. G. and H. A. Simon. 1958. *Organizations.* New York: John Wiley and Sons, Inc.

Marin, V. M. and E. F. Vacha. 1994. Self help strategies and resources among people at risk of homelessness: empirical findings and social services policy. *Social Work* 39(6):649-668.

Marris, P. and M. Rein. 1973. *Dilemmas of social reform.* Chicago: Aldine.

Marston, J. E. 1963. *The Nature of Public Relations.* New York: McGraw-Hill.

Martin, P. Y. and G. G. O'Connor. 1989. *The social environment.* White Plains, NY: Longman.

Maslow, A. H. 1970. *Motivation and personality.* 2d ed. New York: Harper & Row.

Mathieson, T. 1971. *Across organizational boundaries.* Berkeley, CA: Glendessy.

McGee, G. S. and R. T. Crow. 1982. Applicability of assessment center concepts and techniques for managerial selection and development in human service organizations. *Administration in Social Work* 6(1):11-19.

McGowan, B. G. 1974. Case advocacy: A study of the intervention process in child advocacy. Unpublished doctoral dissertation, Columbia University.

McGuire, C. 1995. Personal communication.

McGuire, J. and B. H. Gottieb. 1979. Social support groups among new parents: An experimental study in primary prevention. *Journal of Child Clinical Psychology* 9:111-116.

McIntyre, E. L. G. 1986. Social networks: Potential for practice. *Social Work* 31(6):421-426.

McMurty, S. L. 1985. Secondary prevention of child maltreatment: A review. *Social Work* 30(1):42-48.

Mechanic, D. 1961. Relevance of group atmosphere and attitudes for the rehabilitation of alcoholics. *Quarterly Journal of Studies on Alcohol* 22:634-45.

Mechanic, D. 1974. *Politics, medicine and social service.* New York: John Wiley.

Mechanic, D. 1978. *Medical sociology.* 2d. ed. New York: Free Press.

Mechanic, D. 1980. *Mental health and social policy.* 2d ed. Englewood Cliffs, NJ: *Prentice-Hall.*

Mechanic, D. 1986. The challenge of chronic mental illness: A retrospective and prospective view. *Hospital and Community Psychiatry* 37(9):891-896.

Mechanic, D. 1989. *Mental health and social policy.* 3d. ed. Englewood Cliffs, NJ: *Prentice-Hall.*

Mehr, J. 1980. *Human services: Concepts and intervention strategies.* Boston, MA: Allyn and Bacon.

Meltzer, J. W. 1982. *Respite care: An emerging family support service.* Washington, DC: Center for Study of Social Policy.

Meyer, C. H. 1987. Content and process in social work practice: A new look at old issues. *Social Work* 32(5):401-404.

Meyer, H. J., E. Litwak, E. J. Thomas, and R. Vinter. 1967. Social work and social welfare. In *The uses of sociology,* ed. P. Lazarsfeld, W. H. Sewell, and H. Wilensky. New York: Basic Books.

Middleman, R. R. and G. Goldberg. 1974. *Social service delivery: A structural approach to social work practice.* New York: Columbia University Press.

Miley, K. K., M. O'Melia, and B. L. DuBois. 1995. *Generalist social work practice: An empowering approach.* Needham Heights, MA: Allyn and Bacon.

Minde, K., N. Shosenberg, P. Marton, J. Thompson, J. Ripley, and S. Burns. 1980. Self help groups in a premature nursery–A controlled evaluation. *Journal of Pediatrics* 96:933-940.

Minkoff, K. 1978. A map of chronic mental patient. In *The chronic mental patient*, ed. J. A. Talbott. American Psychiatric Association 9:11-38.

Mintzberg, H. 1973. *The nature of managerial work*. New York: Harper & Row.

Monahan, D. J., V. L. Greene, and P. D. Coleman. 1992. Caregiver support groups: Factors affecting use of services. *Social Work* 37(3):254-260.

Moore, S. T. 1990. A social work practice model of case management: The case management grid. *Social Work* 35(5):444-448.

Moore, S. T. 1992. Case management and the integration of services: How service delivery systems shape case management. *Social Work* 37(5):418-423.

Moos, R. H. 1974a. *Evaluating treatment environments: A social ecological approach*. New York: John Wiley and Sons.

Moos, R. H. 1974b. *The social climate scales: An overview*. Palo Alto. CA: Consulting Psychologists Press.

Moos, R. H. 1976. *The human context: Environmental determinants of behavior*. New York: John Wiley & Sons, Inc.

Moos, R. H. 1979a. *Evaluating educational environments: Procedures, methods, findings, and policy implications*. San Francisco: Jossey-Bass.

Moos, R. H. 1979b. Improving social settings by social climate measurement and feedback. In *Social and psychological research in community settings*, ed. R. Munoz, L. Snowden, and J. Kelly. San Francisco: Jossey-Bass.

Moos, R. H. 1981. *Work environment scale*. Palo Alto, CA: Consulting Psychologists Press.

Moos, R., S. Lemke, and J. Clayton. 1983. Comprehensive assessment of residential programs: A means of facilitating evaluation and change. *Interdisciplinary Topics in Gerontology* 17:69-83.

Moos, R. H. 1984. *Evaluating treatment environments*, New York: John Wiley & Sons.

Moos, R. H. and S. Lemke. 1983. Assessing and improving social-ecological settings. In *Handbook of social intervention*, ed E. Seidman. Beverly Hills, CA: Sage.

Moos, R. H. and S. Lemke. 1984. *Multiphasic environmental assessment procedure*. Palo Alto, CA. Department of Psychiatry, Stanford University, Veterans Administration Hospital.

Morris, R. 1977. Caring for vs. caring about people. *Social Work* 22(5): 353-359.

Morris, R. 1986. *Rethinking social welfare: Why care for the stranger?* Binghamton, NY: Longman.

Morris, R. 1989. Reconceptualizing social work and community. *Social Work* 34:477-478.

Morris, R. and B. Frieden. 1968. *Urban planning and social policy*. New York: Basic Books.

Morris, R. L. and Lescohier. 1978. Service integration: Real vs. illusory solutions to welfare dilemmas. In *The management of human services*, ed. R. S. Saari and Y. Hasenfeld. New York: Columbia University Press.

Morrissey, J. P., R. C. Tessler, and L. L. Farris. 1979. Being seen but not admitted: A note on some neglected aspects of state hospital deinstitutionalization. *American Journal of Orthopsychiatry* 49: 153-156.

Morrissey, J. P. and H. H. Goldman. 1984. Cycles of reform in the care of the chronically mentally ill. *Hospital and Community Psychiatry* 35(8): 785-793.

Motwani, J. K. and G. M. Herring. 1988. Home care for ventilator-dependent persons: A cost-effective, humane public policy. *Health and Social Work* 13(1):20-34.

Moxley, D. P. 1989. *The practice of case management*. Sage Human Service Guides 58. Newbury Park, CA: Sage.

Mulford, C. L. and D. L. Rogers. 1982. Definitions and models. In *Interorganizational coordination: Theory, research and implementation,* ed. D. L. Rogers, D. A. Whetter & Associates. Ames Iowa: Iowa State University Press.

Mutschler, E and R. A. Cnaan. 1985. Success and failure of computerized information systems: Two cases in human service agencies. *Administration in Social Work* 9(1):67-79.

Mutschler, E. and Y. Hasenfeld, Y. 1986. Integrated information systems for social work practice. *Social Work* 31(5):345-349.

National Association of Professional Geriatric Care Managers. 1993. 655 N. Alvernon Way, Suite 108, Tucson, Arizona 85711.

National Institute of Mental Health. 1977. Community Support Section. Request for proposals. No. NIMH-MH-77-0080-0081. Rockville, MD. National Institute of Mental Health.

Netting, F. E. 1992. Case management: Service or symptom. *Social Work* 37(2):160-164.

Netting, F. E. and F. G. Williams. 1989. Establishing interfaces between community and hospital based service systems for the elderly. *Health and Social Work* 14(2):134-139.

Netting, F. E., F. G. Williams, S. Jones-McClinic, and L. Warrick. 1990. Policies to enhance coordination in hospital-based case management programs. *Health and Social Work* 15(1):15-22.

Neugeboren, B. 1957. *Statistical reporting manual.* New Haven, CT: Community Progress Inc.

Neugeboren, B. 1970a. *Psychiatric clinics: A typology of service patterns.* Metuchen, NJ: Scarecrow Press.

Neugeboren, B. 1970b. Opportunity centered social services. *Social Work* 15: 47-52.

Neugeboren, B. 1986. Systemic barriers to education in social administration. *Administration in Social Work* 10(2):1-13.

Neugeboren, B. 1979. Social policy and administration. *Journal of Sociology and Social Welfare* 6(2):168-197.

Neugeboren, B. 1990a. Letter to editor. *Environmental Practice Social Work* 35(4):273-274.

Neugeboren, B. 1990b. Community responsibility for the self- neglectful client. *Journal of Aging and Social Policy* 3(1/2):111- 126.

Neugeboren, B. 1991. *Organization, policy and practice in the human services.* Binghamton, NY: The Haworth Press.

Neugeboren B. 1993. *Organizational influences on management information systems in the human services.* Paper presented at HUSITA 3 International Conference, Maastricht, Netherlands.

Neugeboren, B. 1994. HBSE and the organizational environment as the context for social work practice. Unpublished manuscript, Rutgers School of *Social Work* New Brunswick, NJ.

Neugeboren, R. 1987. *Organizational innovation and change in child welfare: An experimental report and research findings.* Paper presented at N.A.S.W.'s Meeting of the Profession, New Orleans, September.

New York Times, The. 1988. Hiring practices for civil service revamped. June 24, p. 35.

Niefing, T. 1986. Financial impact. In *Chronic illness: Impact and intervention*, ed. I. Lubkin. Boston, MA: Jones and Bartlett.

Nurius, P. S. and W. Hudson. 1988. Computer-based practice: Future dream or current technology *Social Work.* 33(4):357-362.

O'Connor, G. G. 1988. Case management: System and practice. *Social Casework* 69(2):97-106.

Pancost, D. L., P. Parker, and C. Froland. 1983. *Rediscovery of self help.* Beverly Hills, CA: Sage

Panzetta, A. F. 1971. *Community mental health: Myth and reality.* Philadelphia: Lea & Febiger.

Parsons, R. J., S. H. Hernandez, and J. D. Jorgenson. 1988. Integrated practice: A framework for problem solving. *Social Work* 33(5):417-421.

Patti, R. 1974. Limits and prospects of internal advocacy. *Social Casework* 55(9):537-545.

Patti, R. 1980. Internal advocacy and human service practitioners: An exploratory study. In *Change from within: Humanizing human service organizations*, ed. H. Resnick and R. Patti, 287-301. Philadelphia: Temple Press.

Patti, R. 1983. *Social welfare administration: Managing social programs in a developmental context.* Englewood Cliffs: Prentice-Hall.

Patti, R. J. and M. J. Austin. 1977. Socializing the direct service practitioner in the ways of supervisory management. *Administration in Social Work* 1(3):167-180.

Patti, R. J., J. Poertner, and C. A. Rapp (eds.) *Managing for service effectiveness in social welfare organizations.* New York: The Haworth Press.

Pattison, E. M. 1973. Social system psychotherapy. *American Journal of Psychotherapy*, 18:396-409.

Pecora, P. J. and M J. Austin. 1987. *Managing human services personnel.* Newbury Park, CA: Sage.

Pelton, L. H. (ed.) 1981. *The social context of child abuse and neglect.* New York: Human Science Press.

Pelton, L. H. 1982. Personalistic attributions and client perspectives in child welfare cases: Implications for service delivery. In *Basic processes in helping relationships*, ed. T. A. Wills. New York: Academic Press.

Perlman, R. and V. A. Gurin. 1972. *Community organization and social planning*. New York: John Wiley & Sons.

Perlmutter, F., S. Heinemann, and L. Yudin. 1974. Public welfare clients and community mental health centers. *Public Welfare* Spring, 39-42.

Perrow, C. 1976. *The centralized decentralized bureaucracy form of control*. Paper presented at 71 St. Annual Meeting of the American sociological Association, New York.

Phillips, B. A., B. Dimsdale, and E. Taft. 1985. An information system for the social casework agency: A model and case study. In *Managing finances, personnel, and information in human services*. Vol. 2 of *Social Administration: The Management of the Social Services*. 2d edition. New York: The Haworth Press.

Pilisuk, M. and S. H. Parks. 1988. Caregivers: When families need help. *Social Work* 33(5):436-440.

Pincus, A. and A. Minihan. 1973. *Social work practice: Model and method*. Itasca, IL: Peacock.

Pines, A. M. and E. Aronson. 1981. *Burnout: From tedium to personal growth*. New York: Macmillan

Pines, A. M. and C. Maslach. 1978. Characteristics of staff burnout in mental health settings. *Hospital and Community Psychiatry* 4:233-237.

Poertner, J and C. Rapp. 1980. Information system design in foster care. *Social Work* 25:114-119.

Poertner, J. and C. Rapp. 1985. Purchase of service and accountability: Will they ever meet. *Administration in Social Work* 9(1):57-66.

Poole, D. L. 1987. Social policy and mental illness. *Health and Social Work* 12(40):246-249.

Popple, P. R. 1984. Negotiation: A critical skill for social work administrators. *Administration in Social Work* 8(2):1-12.

Prager, E. and D. Shnit. 1985. Organizational environment and case outcome decisions for elderly clientele: A view from Israel. *Administration in Social Work* 9(4):49-62.

President's Commission on Mental Health. 1978. *Task Panel Reports*. Vols. 2-4. Washington, DC: Government Printing Office.

Proctor, E. K., N. R. Voster, and E. A. Sirles. 1993. The social environment context of child clients. An empirical exploration. *Social Work* 38(3):256-262.

Rapp, C. A. 1984. Information performance, and the human service manager of the 1980s: Beyond housekeeping. *Administration in Social Work* 8(2):69-80.

Rapp, C. A. and S. Anderson. 1975. Improving direct service workers informatin system performance. In *Child welfare information systems*, ed. M. Taber et al. Urbania, IL: University of Illinois.

Rapp, C. A. and R. Chamberlain. 1985. Case management services for the chronically mentally ill. *Social Work* 30(5):417-422.

Rapp, C. A and J. Poertner. 1986. The design of data-based management reports. *Administration in Social Work* 10(4):53-64.

Rapp, C. A. and J. Poertner. 1987. Moving clients center stage through the use of client outcomes. *Administration in Social Work* 11(3/4):23-38.

Rapp, C. A. and J. Poertner. 1992. *Social administration: A client centered approach*. White Plains, NY: Longman.

Rauktis, M. E. and G. F. Koeske. 1994. Maintaining social worker morale: When supportive supervision is not enough. *Administration in Social Work* 18(1):39-60.

Ray, O. and C. Ksir. 1987. *Drugs, society, & human behavior.* St. Louis: Times Mirror/Mosby.

Reich, C. 1970. *Greening of America: How the youth revolution is trying to make America liveable.* New York: Random House.

Reid, W. J. 1965. Inter-agency coordination in delinquency preventon and control. In *Social welfare institutions*, ed. M. Zald. New York: John Wiley & Sons.

Reid, W. and C. Beard. 1980. An evaluation of in-service training in public welfare setting. *Administration in Social Work* 4(1): 71-85.

Reid, W. J. and P. Hanrahan. 1982. Recent evaluations of social work: Grounds for optimism. *Social Work* 27(4).

Reid, W. J. 1987. Service effectiveness and the social agency. *Administration in Social Work* 11(3/4): 41-58.

Rein, M. and R. Morris. 1969. Goals, strategies and structures for community change. In *Readings in community organization practice*, ed. R. Kramer and H. Specht. Englewood Cliffs, NJ: Prentice-Hall.

Rein, M. 1969. Research design and social policy in distress in the city. In *Distress to the city*, ed. W. Ryan. Cleveland: Case Western Reserve.

Rein, M. 1970. Social work in search for a radical perspective. *Social Work* 15(2):13-28.

Rice, D. and M. Hodgson. 1981. Social and economic implications in the United States. In *U. S. Public Health Service. Vital Statistics*. Series 3, No. 20. Department of Health and Services. Publication No. PHS-81-1404. Washington, DC: U. S. Government Printing Office.

Richardson, J. L., J. W. Graham, and D. R. Shelton. 1989. Social environment and adjustment after Laryngetomy. *Health and Social Work* 14(4):283-292.

Richmond, M. E. 1922. *What is social casework?* New York: Russell Sage.

Rogers-Warren, A. and S. F. Warren. (eds.) 1977. *Ecological perspectives in behavior analysis*. Baltimore: University Park Press.

Rose, S. P. 1992. Case management: An advocacy/empowerment design. *Social work and case management*. New York: Longman.

Rosengren, W. R. 1967. Structure, policy, and style: Strategies for organizational control. *Administration Science Quarterly* 12: 140-164.

Rosenthal, M. G. 1994. Single mothers in Sweden: Work and welfare in the welfare state. *Social Work* 39(3):270-279.

Rothman, J. 1979. Three models of community organization practice. In *Strategies of community organization*. F. M. Cox et al. 3d ed. Itasca, IL: F. E. Peacock.

Rothman, J. 1980. *Using research in organizations*. Beverly Hills, CA: Sage.

Rothman, J. 1991. A model for case management: Toward empirically based practice. *Social Work* 36(6):520-528.

Rothman, J. 1994. *Practice with highly vulnerable clients. Case management and community based service*. Englewood Cliffs, NJ: Prentice-Hall.

Rubin, A. 1985. Practice effectivensss: More grounds for optimism. *Social Work* 38(6):469-476.

Rubin, A. 1992. Is case management effective for people with serious mental illness? A research review. *Health and Social Work* 17(2):138-150.

Rubin, A. and P. J. Johnson. 1984. Direct practice of entering M.S.W. students. *Journal of Education for Social Work* 20:5-16.

Ryan, F. J. 1958. Further observations on competitive ability in athletics. In *Psychosocial problems in college men*, ed. B. Wedge. New Haven: Yale University Press.

Ryan, W. 1971. *Blaming the victim.* New York: Random House.

Salem, D. A., E. Seiderman, and J. Rappaport. 1988. Community treatment of the mentally ill: The promise of mutual-help organizations. *Social Work* 33(5):403-408.

Sanborn, C. J. (ed.). 1983. *Case management in mental health services.* New York: The Haworth Press.

Sauser, W. I. 1980. Evaulating employee performance: Needs, problems, and possible solutions. *Public Personnel Management* 9(1):11-18.

Saxton, P. 1991. Comments on Social Work and the Psychotherapies. *Social Service Review* 65(2):314-317.

Schachter, S. 1959. *The psychology of affiliation.* Palo Alto, CA: Stanford University Press.

Scheff, T. J. 1968. Societal reaction to deviance: Ascriptive elements in the psychiatric screening of mental patients in a midwestern state. In *The mental patient: Studies in the sociology of deviance*, ed. S. P. Spitzer and N. K. Denzin. New York: McGraw-Hill.

Schilling II, R. F. 1987. Limitations of social support. *Social Service Review* 61(1):19-31.

Schilling, R. F., S. P. Schinke, and R. A. Weatherly. 1988. Service trends in a conservative era: Social workers discover the past. *Social Work* 33(1):5-10.

Schlesinger, E. G. 1985. *Health care social work: Concepts and strategies.* St. Louis: Times Mirror/Mosby.

Schmidt, F. and H. N. Weiner. 1966. *Public relations in health and welfare.* New York: Columbia University Press.

Schneider, R. L. 1978. Behavior outcomes for administration majors. *Journal of Social Work Education* 14(3):98-102.

Schneider, R. L. and N. Sharon. 1982. Representation of social work agencies: New definition, special issues, and practice model. *Administration in Social Work* 6(1):59-68.

Schopler, J. H. and M. J. Galinsky. 1993. Support groups are open systems: A model for practice and research. *Health and Social Work* 18(13):195-207.

Schriver, J. M. 1987. Harry Lurie's critique: Person and environment in early casework practice. *Social Service Review* 61(3):514-532.

Schwartz, E. E. 1977. Macro social work: A practice in search of some theory. *Social Service Review* 51:210-218.

Schwartz, W. 1969. Private troubles and public issues: One social work job or two. *1969 Social welfare forum*. New York: Columbia University Press.

Seebohm Report. 1968. *Report of the committee on local authority and allied personal social services*. Cmnd. 3703, HMSO.

Segal, S. P. and J. Baumohl. 1980. Engaging the disengaged: Proposals on madness and vagrancy. *Social Work* 25(5):358-365.

Segal, S. P., J. Baumohl, and L. H. Liése. 1993.

Segal, S. P., C. Silverman, and T. Temkon. 1993. Empowerment and self help agency practice for people with mental disabilities. *Social Work* 38(6):705-712.

Segal, S. P., D. J. Vandervort, and L. H. Liése. 1993. Residential status and the physical health of a mentally ill population. *Health and Social Work* 18(3):208-214.

Select Committee on Aging. U. S. House of Representatives (Stone, R.). 1987. *Exploding the myths: Caregiving in America*. (One hundredth Congress, First Session. Comm. Pub. No. 99-611) Washington, DC: U. S. Government Printing Office.

Seltzer, M. M., J. Ivry, and L. C. Lichfield. 1992. Family members as case manager. Partnership between formal and informal support networks. In *Case management and social work practice*, ed. S. M. Rose. New York: Longman.

Selznick, P. 1957. *Leadership in administration*. Evanston, IL: Harper & Row.

Shaw, S. and T. Borkman. 1990. *Social model of alcohol recovery: An environmental approach*. Burbank, CA: Bridge Focus Inc.

Silverman, P. R. 1980. *Mutual help groups: Organization and development*. Beverly Hills, CA: Sage.

Silverman, P. R. et al. (eds.) 1974. *Helping each other in widowhood.* New York: Health Sciences.

Simon, E. P., N. Showers, S. Blumenfield, G. Holden, and X. Wu. 1995. Delivery of home care services after discharge: What really happens. *Health and Social Work* 20(1):5-14.

Simons, R. L. 1985. Inducements as an approach to exercising influence. *Social Work* 30(6):469-476.

Siporin, M. 1975. *Introduction to social work practice.* New York: Macmillan.

Slavin, S. 1985. Introduction to information, computers, and management. In *Managing finances, personnel, and information in human services.* Vol. 2 of *Social Administration: The management of the social services.* 2d. ed. New York: The Haworth Press.

Smith, M. O. 1988. Acupuncture treatment for crack: Clinical survey of 1500 patients treated. *American Journal of Acupuncture* 16(3):241-246.

Sosa, R., J. Kennell, M. Klaus, S. Robertson,, and J. Urrutia. 1980. The effect of a supportive companion on perinatal problems, length of labor, and mother-infant interaction. *New England Journal of Medicine* 303:597-600.

Sosin, M. R. 1990. Decentralizing the social service system: A reassessment. *Social Service Review* 64(4):617-636.

Specht, H. 1985 Managing professional interpersonal interactions. *Social Work* 30:225-230.

Specht, H. J. 1988. *New directions for social work practice.* Englewood Cliffs, NJ: Prentice-Hall.

Specht, H. and Courtney, M. 1994. *Unfaithful angels: How social work has abandoned its mission.* New York: Free Press.

Speck, R. V. and C. Attneave. 1993. *Family networks.* New York: Pantheon.

Speck, R. V. and U. Rueveni. 1973. *Family networks.* New York: Pantheon.

Spitzer, T. 1980. *Psychobattery: A chronicle of psychotherapeutic abuse.* Clifton, NJ: Human Press.

Stanton, A. H. and M. Schwartz. 1954. *The mental hospital: A study of institutional participation in psychiatric illness and treatment.* New York: Basic Books.

Stein, L. I. 1979. *Community support systems for the long-term patient. New directions for mental health services.* No. 2. San Francisco: Jossey-Bass.

Stein, L. I., M. Test, and A. J. Marx. 1975. Alternative to the hospital: A controlled study. *American Journal of Psychiatry* 132:517-522.

Stein, L. I. and M. A. Test. 1980. Alternatives to mental hospital treatment. *Archives of General Psychiatry* 37:392-397.

Steiner, R. 1977. *Managing the human service organization.* Beverly Hills, CA: Sage.

Strauss, A. and Glaser. 1975. *Chronic illness and the quality of life.* St. Louis: Mosby.

Strauss, A. J. et al. 1984. *Chronic illness and the quality of life.* 2d ed. St. Louis: Mosby.

Strauss, A. J. and J. M. Corbin. 1988. *Shaping a new health care system.* San Francisco: Jossey-Bass.

Strauss, A., S. Fagerhaugh, B. Suczek, and C. Wiener. 1985. *The social organization of medical work.* Chicago: University of Chicago Press.

Streeter, C. L., M. W. Sherraden, D. F. Gellespie, and M. J. Zakour. 1986. Curriculum development in interorganizational coordination. *Journal of Social Work Education* 22(1):32-40.

Stroul, B. A. 1986. *Models of community support services: Approaches to helping persons with long-term mental illness.* Boston, MA: Center for Psychiatric Rehabilitation.

Stuen, C. and A. Monk. 1991. Discharge planning: The impact of Medicare's perspective payment on elderly patients. *Journal of Gerontological Social Work* 15:145-165.

Sullivan, W. P. 1992. Reclaiming the community: The strengths perspective and deinstitutionalization. *Social Work* 37(3):204-209.

Talbott, J. A. 1981. *The chronically mentally ill.* New York: Human Sciences Press.

Taylor, M. S. 1987. The effects of feedback on the behavior of organizational personnel. *Administration in Social Work* 11(3/4): 191-204.

Teare, R. 1981. *Social work practice in a public welfare setting.* New York: Praeger.

Tedeschi, J. T. and P. Rosenfeld. 1980. Communication in bargaining and negotiation. In *Persuasion: New direction in theory and research*, M. Roloff and G. Miller ed. Beverly Hills, CA: Sage.

Thomas, C. H. 1983. Social model. *Social Work* 26(4):271-273.

Thomas, D. T. 1983. *The making of community work*. London: George Allen Unwin.

Thomas, D. and H. Shaftoe. 1974. Does casework need a neighborhood orientation? *Social Work Today* 5:483-486.

Thomas, E. 1959. Role conceptions and organizational size. *American Sociological Review* 24:30-37.

Thurz, D. and J. L. Vigilante (eds.). 1978. *Reaching people: The structure of neighborhood services*. Vol. 3. *Social services delivery systems*. Berverly Hills, CA: Sage.

Tobin, S. and R. Kulys. 1981. The family in the institutionalization of the elderly. *Journal of Social Issues* 37:145-157.

Todd, D. M. 1980. *Social networks, psychosocial adaptation, and preventive/developmental interventions: The support development workshop*. Paper presented at the meeting of the American Psychological Association, Montreal.

Tolson, E. R. 1994. *Generalist practice: A task centered approach*. New York: Columbia University Press.

Tonnies, F. 1957. *Community and society*. Translated and edited C. P. Loomis. Michigan: Michigan State University Press.

Torczyner, J. and A. Pare. 1979. The influence of environmental factors on foster care. *Social Service Review* 53(3):358-377.

Toseland, R. W., W. J. Reid, and C. D. Garvin. 1990. Long term effectiveness of peer-led and professionally led support groups for caregivers. *Social Service Review* 64(2):308-327.

Toseland, R. W. and L. Hacker. 1985. Social workers use of self help groups as a resource for clients. *Social Work* 30:232-237.

Toseland, R. W., C. M. Rossiter, and M. S. Labreque. 1989. The effectiveness of two kinds of support groups for caregivers. *Social Service Review* 63(3):415-432.

Toseland, R. W., C. M. Rossiter, T. Peak, and G. C. Smith. 1990. Comparative effectiveness of individual and group interventions to support family caregivers. *Social Work* 35(3):209-219.

Treas, J. 1981. The great American fertility debate: Generational balance and support of the aged. *The Gerontologist*, 17 98-103.

Tripody, T., P. Fellin, and I. Epstein. 1978. *Differential social program evaluation.* Itasca, IL: Peacock.

U.S. Dept. of Health, Education and Welfare. 1979. *Healthy people: Surgeon General's report on health promotion and disease prevention.* Washington, DC: Government Printing Office.

U.S. General Accounting Office. 1978. *Information and referral for people needing human services.* Washington, DC: Comptroller Generals report to Congress, HRD-77-134.

Vachon, M. L. S. 1987. *Occupational stress in the care of the critically ill, the dying, and the bereaved.* New York: Harper & Row.

Vaughn, C. E. and J. P. Leff. 1976. The measurement of expressed emotion in the families of psychiatric patients. *British Journal of Social and Clinical Psychology* 15:157-165.

Videka-Sherman, L. 1988. Metanalysis of research in social work practice in mental health. *Social Work* 33(4):325-337.

Vladeck, B. 1983. Two steps forward, one back: The changing agenda of long term home care reform. *Pride Institute Journal of Long-Term Home Care* 2:1-7.

Vladeck, B. 1985. The static dynamics of long term health policy. In *The Health Agenda,* ed. M. Levine. Washington, DC: American Enterprise Institute.

Vosler, R. V. 1990. Assessing family access to basic resources: An essential component of social work practice. *Social Work* 35(5):434-441.

Walker, R. 1972. The ninth panacea: Program evaluation. *Evaluation* 1:45-53.

Walsh, J. 1988. Social workers as family educators. *Social Work* 33(2):138-141.

Walters, J. and B. Neugeboren. 1995. Collaboration between mental health organizations and religious institutions. *Psychosocial Rehabilitation Journal* 19(2):51-57.

Walz, T., G. Willenberg, and L. DeMoll. 1974. Environmental design. *Social Work* 19(1):38-47.

Warheit, G. J., R. A. Bell, and J. J. Schwab. 1978. *Planning for change: Need assessment approaches.* Washington, DC: National Institute of Mental Health.

Warren, D. I. 1981. *Helping networks*. Notre Dame, IN: Notre Dame Press.

Warren, R. 1963. *The community in America*. Chicago: Rand McNally.

Webb, A. and G. Wistow. 1987. *Social work, social care and social planning: The personal social services since Seebohm*. New York: Longman.

Weeden, J. P., R. J. Newcomer, and T. O. Byerts. 1986. *Housing and shelter for frail and non-frail elders: Current options and future directions. In Housing an aging society: Issues, alternatives, and policy*, ed. R. J. Newcomer, M. P. Lawton, and T. O. Byerts. 181-187. New York: Van Nostrand.

Weick, A., C. Rapp, W. P. Sullivan, and W. Kisthardt. 1989. A strengths perspective for social work practice. *Social Work* 34: 350-354.

Weiner, M. E. 1990. Human services management: Analysis and applications. 2nd edition. Belmont, CA: Wadsworth.

Weinman, B. and R. J. Kleiner. 1978. The impact of community living and community member intervention on the adjustment of the chronic mental patient. In *Alternatives to mental hospital treatment*, ed. L. I. Stein and M. A. Test. New York: Plenum Press. 139-159.

Weirich, T. W. 1985. The design of information systems. In *Managing finances, personnel, and information in human services*. Vol. 2 of *Social Administration: The Management of the Social Services*. 2d ed. New York: The Haworth Press 315-329.

Weisenfeld, A. R. and H. M. Weiss. 1979. A mental health consultation program for beauticians. Professional Psychology 10:786-792.

Weisman, A. 1976. Industrial social services: Linkage technology. *Social Casework* 57:50-54.

Weisman, A. 1987. Linkage in direct practice. In *Encyclopedia of Social Work* Vol. II. Washington, DC: NASW.

Weiss, C. H. 1972. *Evaluative research: Methods of assessing program effectiveness*. New York: Prentice-Hall.

Weissman, H. 1977. Clients, staff, and researchers: Their role in management information systems. *Administration in Social Work* 1(1):43-51.

Weissman, H. 1987. Planning for client feedback: Content and context. *Administration in Social Work* 11(3/4):205-220.

Weissman, H., I. Epstein, and A. Savage. 1983. *Agency based social work: Neglected aspects of clinical practice.* Phildelphia: Temple Press.

Wells, L. M. and C. Singer. 1985. A model for linking networks in social work practice with the institutionalized elderly. *Social Work* 30(4):318-322.

Westman, D. P. 1991. *Whistleblowing: The law of retaliatory discharge.* Washington, DC: BNA Books.

Wetzel, J. 1978. The work environment and depression: Implications for intervention. In *Toward human Dignity: Social work in practice*, ed. J. Hanks. Washington, DC: National Association of Social Workers.

White, M. 1987. Case management. In *Encylopedia of aging.* New York: Springer-Verlag. 93-96.

Whittaker, J. K. 1974. *Social treatment.* Chicago: Aldine.

Whittaker, J. K., J. Garbarino, and associates. 1983. *Social support networks: Informal helping in the human services.* New York: Aldine.

Whittaker, J. K., S. P. Schinke, and L. D. Gilchrist. 1986. The ecological paradigm in child, youth, and family services: Implications for policy and practice. *Social Service Review* 60(4):483-503.

Wiegerink, R. and K. J. W. Pelosi (eds.) 1979. *Developmental disabilities: The D.D. movement.* Baltimore: Paul Brooks.

Wiehe, V. R. 1980. Current practice in performance appraisal. *Administration in Social Work* 4(3):1-12.

Wilbur, C. S. 1983. The Johnson and Johnson program. *Preventive Medicine* 12:672-681.

Wilensky, H. and C. Lebeaux. 1958. *Industrial society and social welfare.* New York: Russell Sage.

Williams, W. 1975. Implementation, analysis and assessment. *Policy Analysis* 1:15-48.

Wilson, J. Q. (ed.) 1966. *Urban renewal: The record and the controversy.* Cambridge: MIT. Press.

Wintersteen, R. T. 1986. Rehabilitating the chronically mentally ill: Social work's claim to leadership. *Social Work* 31(5):332-337.

Wittman, M. 1978. Application of knowledge about prevention to health and mental health practice. In *Social work in health care*, ed. N. F. Bracht. New York: The Haworth Press.

Wolfensberger, W. 1972. *Normalization.* Toronto: National Institute of Mental Retardation.

Wolfensberger, W. and L. Glenn. 1975. Program analysis of service systems. *Handbook and Field Manual.* 3d ed. Toronto: National Institute on Mental Retardation.

Wolk, J. L., W. P. Sullivan, and D. J. Hartmann. 1994. The managerial nature of case management. *Social Work* 39(2):152-159.

Wolowitz, D. 1983. Clients rights in a case management system. In *Case management in mental health services*, ed. C. J. Sandhorn. 81-90. New York: The Haworth Press.

Wood. J. B. and C. L. Estes. 1988. Medicalization of community services for the elderly. *Health and Social Work* 13(1):35-42.

Wood, G. G. and R. Middleman. 1989. *The structural approach to direct practice in social work: A textbook for students and front-line practitioners.* New York: Columbia Press.

York, R. O. and H. Henley. 1986. Perceptions of bureaucracy. *Administration in Social Work* 10(1):3-15.

Zald, M. N. 1965. *Organizations as polities: Concepts for the analysis of community organization agencies.* Office of Juvenile Delinquency and Youth Development, Department of Health, Education and Welfare.

Name Index

Subject Index

Page numbers followed by a "t" indicate tables.